Today's Students, Tomorrow's Doctors

Reflections from the wards

Kathy Feest
Associate Dean and Director of the Foundation School Severn Institute, Bristol
Special Advisor to Foundation Programmes for Modernising Medical Careers
(MMC), London

and

Karen Forbes
Macmillan Professorial Teaching Fellow
United Bristol Healthcare Trust and University of Bristol

Forewords by

Sir Kenneth Calman
Vice-Chancellor and Warden
Durham University

Dr Lynn Calman
School of Nursing, Midwifery and Social Work
University of Manchester

and

Professor Rita Charon
Professor of Clinical Medicine, College of Physicians and Surgeons of Columbia University, New York

D0165135

Radcliffe Publishing
Oxford • Seattle

Radcliffe Publishing Ltd
18 Marcham Road
Abingdon
Oxon OX14 1AA
United Kingdom

**W
18
F295t
2006**

www.radcliffe-oxford.com
Electronic catalogue and worldwide online ordering facility.

British Library Cataloguing in Publication Data

A catalogue record for this book is available from the British Library.

ISBN-10: 1 84619 078 9
ISBN-13: 978 1 84619 078 0

Typeset by Lapiz Digital Services, Chennai
Printed and bound by TJ International Ltd, Padstow, Cornwall

Contents

Foreword

We approached this book with no preconceived ideas: we were delighted, surprised and at times concerned. Delighted because of the issues raised and the sophisticated ways in which students responded to the challenges; surprised at the range of issues raised and the obvious importance of relationships in the clinical setting; finally concerned at some of the attitudes which were commented on, especially of senior staff, and on the adequacy of preparation for house officer posts.

This book presents the reflections of a series of medical students during their two weeks shadowing the house officer they were to take over from and become a 'real doctor' with responsibilities and relationships to manage. It was a joy to read, full of hope and inspiration. It is clear that the students learned a great deal – about themselves as much as anything – and the people with whom they would work. They are very mature essays, full of sensitivity and insight, and they show the power of narrative in setting out feelings and emotions. The stories highlight students' first experiences of juggling the priorities of the system and the needs of individual patients. They reminded us of our first days of responsibility, the first proper thanks from a patient or a family and the first present as a student – a delicious curry brought into the ward in the pot ready for heating up.

They illustrate clearly the sense of community that exists in some places and not in others. The importance of role models is also clear in the statements made about those whom they will succeed. They notice and focus on the small issues: the importance of a smile, of being organised, of getting on with others, of the skill required to get an x-ray out-of-hours or in a hurry, and the way they were treated by qualified staff.

There are several disturbing episodes where the team was not functioning well, where the senior medical person was feared, if not loathed, and in some cases how poor the communication was, especially in the issue of breaking bad news. These must be the most disturbing aspects of the essays; that at the start of the 21st century some doctors still behave in a manner which is just not acceptable.

The relationships with nurses and professionals allied to medicine are also of interest and there are lessons to be learned. The accounts of students highlight important examples of successful and unsuccessful interprofessional communication. Other professionals can be important role models for junior medical staff; the students often commented on situations where they had learned from the experience, values and attitudes of others.

Patients and relatives were also highlighted as partners in care in these accounts and the students describe their opportunities to discuss difficult decisions and news with them and reflect on what can be learned from getting it right and sometimes getting it wrong.

A particular issue that struck a chord, which elsewhere we have referred to as the 'my mother principle', was the sensitivity of the students in recognising the importance of people. If it was your mother, child, brother, how would you want them to be cared for? These young people could see the value of caring for people, which was humbling to read. They clearly learned from this experience.

So what lessons can be learned from these essays? First, they are worth reading and the students themselves learned from the experiences. Second, there are implications for the medical course itself. Most were prepared for the tasks ahead, but in some areas, notably in dealing with very ill and dying patients, they needed more experience. They recognised the importance of being organised and being able to cope with a rapidly changing environment. One of the most important lessons for the students was that the knowledge and skills (for example, taking an arterial blood gas, filling in forms) which were the primary concern of students when they started their shadowing experience seemed insignificant when faced with the human skills needed to deal with emergency situations, human tragedy and loss. Perhaps more could be done to give additional experience of this.

In relating to other professional groups the opportunity to shadow and work with other professionals, particularly nurses, allowed students to gain an insight into the roles and responsibilities of others and to understand that everyone, including patients, has competing pressures and needs. Good team working and communication allow these difficulties to be resolved successfully. There is a need to help senior staff recognise the importance of supervision of juniors and the ways in which mentoring and feedback on performance can assist the functioning of the whole team. Some senior staff clearly need more help on the question of communication skills and it is disappointing that such problems still exist, as perceived by a group of bright, intelligent medical students about to embark on a career in medicine. They have learned from such behaviour.

This book is inspirational and should be read by all who have any part to play in the education of doctors.

Sir Kenneth Calman
Vice-Chancellor and Warden
Durham University

Dr Lynn Calman
School of Nursing, Midwifery and Social Work
University of Manchester
September 2006

Foreword

These essays written by final-year medical students at Bristol University Medical School tell more than they seem to tell – about themselves, about the enterprise of medical education, and about the effective care of the sick. The students were asked to write the essays during a newly inaugurated educational effort called 'Shadowing' that orients medical students to their future tasks as hospital house officers. Written by the students at the end of a two-week period of accompanying the PRHOs whose jobs they will assume very soon thereafter, these reflective accounts capture early and profoundly formative clinical experiences.

Grouped into sections like 'Relationships', 'Working in the system' and 'Death', the essays reflect a fresh calculus of sickness and duty. Not only, now, are students seeing and learning about such diseases as end-stage colon cancer and rapidly progressive dementia, but they have some capacity to act on behalf of the patients who host these diseases and, even, are burdened with and buoyed by the expectations of doctors and nurses and patients and patients' families that indeed they will do something for the sick person.

I am first of all impressed with the emotional valence of these writings. They reflect the students' interior states of sadness, empathy, and awe as they bear witness to patients' suffering. About a 51-year-old woman learning her colon cancer was inoperable, a student writes:

> She never moved her gaze from the bearer of bad news. ... Her life had changed in a second. Was she still listening to him? How could she take all this in? 'Advanced cancer' ... 'extensive disease' ... 'some chemotherapy might help' ... 'the oncologist will come and see you' ... *'I wish I was standing here telling you that I have removed all the cancer'* ... I looked around the characters in this scene, putting myself into each person's shoes in turn. How was the patient so gentle and accepting? Why wasn't she angry? Her husband stared at the floor. I looked at her father who was looking at me. ... Could he see my genuine sadness, coming from that part of the heart so deep that it must actually be in the stomach, because it was making me feel sick. His daughter was the same age as my mother. (p. 91)

The student recognises the efforts of the surgeon to convey this horrible news gently, the shocking disbelief and loss experienced by the patient and her family, and the student's own in part corporeal experience of the situation. A sadness so deep it feels it comes from the gut, this feeling ties the student intimately to this family, in part through the agency of an associative recognition tying in the health of her own mother. What impresses me beyond the representational accuracy of this emotional reflection is the student's disciplined imagination in adopting each person's perspective by turn. What a professionally sophisticated accomplishment for a student, one which we hope to encourage and not to dismiss.

The next thing that strikes me about these reflections is how *young* their authors seem to me. It is hard for me to believe that they have been in medical school already for four or five years, so unused do they seem to be to the experience – or even the notion – of being clinically useful. 'Investigation ordering, form filling and drug chart adjusting are all skills I am yet to be proficient in. I perform them with the slow awkward concentration of a middle-aged man being taught to knit' (p. 8). Besides being extraordinarily good writing, these sentences convey the clumsy humiliation of someone doing something alien to his station. Disoriented by doing doctorly things, the students face the gulf between the students they are and the doctors they yearn to be. 'Throughout medical school you usually feel that you are in someone's way, that you're just someone who clutters up ward rounds or clinics and takes up valuable time because you have to be taught' (p. 21). Well. Such comments are marvellously useful to us faculty, exposing a lesion in our educational system that does not feed back to students what, all along, they teach us and donate to us from their own fresh and idealistic perspectives.

For they teach us tremendous amounts about who we are and what we do. In the introduction to this collection, the editors point to the anthropological belief that 'medicine is an exquisitely perceptive indicator of the essential cultural characteristics of any period' (p. 1). To draw out this notion, what we are asking young students to do is to write what amount to anthropologists' field notes that comment on the bizarre rituals of this strange culture they are newly privy to. This interloper stance enables the students to perceive the oddness and deficiencies of the hospital – its rigid hierarchy, its sometimes bad manners, its rusty procedures. One student describes work rounds:

> The bit that really got to me was going to see a rather frail elderly lady who had just had an endoscopy for dysphagia. An oesophageal cancer was discovered and an attempt to place an oesophageal stent had been made at the initial endoscopy but was unsuccessful.
>
> Instead of ordering away the unnecessary onlookers from the bed and breaking the news of her cancer slowly, quietly and gently, the surgeon proceeded to tell her that 'We have found a malignant growth in your oesophagus and we tried to deploy a stent to relieve your dysphagia but it failed to deploy properly so we are going to try again but with a longer Flamingo this time. Any questions? No? OK, good, see you tomorrow'. And bear in mind that this was with the curtains open, 10 people observing and no relatives with the patient. I was horrified at this and felt desperately sorry for the elderly lady. No doubt all she would have understood of the surgeon's statement was that she had cancer and that the doctors' efforts to relieve her symptoms had failed. How frightening for her! (p. 32)

Not only for the sake of this student but for the sake of medicine must we safeguard or at least learn from this impression, this clairvoyance born of freshness of vision and purity of motive. Indeed, this citation helps us to identify the ideal audience for these writings. *All* of us in medicine – doctors, medical educators, nurses, hospital administrators – must read and take seriously the charges levelled by these reflections. These students see what we, having gone native, cannot see. Only once we see reality as refracted through the students' gaze can we appreciate how we might improve our systems of care.

Although there are indeed stories here of medical failures and lapses, medicine's caring powers predominate in the students' writing. The student-writers see and value their supervisors' models of attentive and effective care. One student learns about silence and apology in the practice of medicine:

> I think we need more of the wordless in our lives. We need more still-ness, more of a sense of wonder, a feeling for the mystery of life. ... [My PRHO] knew how to say 'I'm sorry' and he said it well. ... The realisation came to me when we went to see a patient with a bed sore, who had been given an air pressure mattress. She wasn't happy with this and was crying out to anyone who would listen to ask the doctors to change it back. We went to see her to explain. He listened to her for what seemed like a long while. My first red flag that something was unusual was that he was absolutely silent whilst listening to her. No pacifying 'hmmms', no dismissive 'yes, I knows'. All he did was listen to her while looking directly at her, and then say, with the most gen-tle caring tone I've ever heard, 'I'm sorry'. He paused for a bit to let her absorb that apology, and then continued to explain why she had to have the mattress. Watching him felt like one of those surreal moments in time, perhaps akin to that moment people talk about before blacking out or having a fit ... things go quiet, things slow down ... your vision becomes tunnelled and absolutely focused ... and then you come to. He did it again while I was shadowing him and, again, it felt odd to watch. (I know now that 'odd' feeling was the feeling of being really moved.)
>
> I realised at that moment that on the whole, when I apologise to patients, to consultants, to other people, I'm apologising for myself, for my lack of skills or knowledge, for my error in judgement. My PRHO made me see that my focus is completely misguided. When I apolo-gise, the focus is about me. When he apologises, the focus is on the other person who is suffering. That is the way it should be. (pp. 35–6)

Now, this is an extraordinary stretch of writing. Not only is it well crafted, it seamlessly unites the writer's detailed representation of an external event, a cog-nitive interpretation of the event, the writer's interior affective experiences dur-ing the event, and then the synthesised result of having undergone all this. This is autobiographical insight at its most powerful, for it leads to transformative growth and true learning.

The architects of this learning exercise and their students have accomplished a great deal. By encouraging the use of reflective writing, the faculty have donated sturdy methods of life-long learning to their students. Writing – especially, it seems, in clinical settings – grants us access to that which we know without real-ising we know it. Such writing unites clinician-writers with patients, for the writ-ing is inevitably a braiding of biography of patient and autobiography of clinician. As a dividend, this writing illuminates our professional enterprise, shining odd and fruitful light on what might pass as routine or ordinary or below notice. All that is involved in the Shadowing course – the exposure of students to their soon-to-be-selves, the requirement that they commit some of their experiences to writing, and then the serious attention to the resultant texts – cohere toward fundamental growth for students and a liberating humility and joy for their teachers. In the words of one student:

> If this shadowing course has taught me anything, it has made me realise how important, even as a junior, our time and effort is to patients, and how, ultimately, respecting their individuality, and helping them confront their mortality by looking into their eyes and confronting your own, makes you a far better doctor than efficiency with blood forms ever will. (p. 102)

These texts give me great and glad hope that our doctors of the future will be efficient with the forms of medicine as well as courageous in braving their contact with the ill, with the dying, with the humans who confront them evermore seeking care, seeking comfort, seeking their full capacity to heal.

Rita Charon
Professor of Clinical Medicine
College of Physicians and Surgeons of Columbia University
New York, NY
September 2006

Preface

The narratives presented here are 'reflective accounts' written by final year medical students from Bristol University between 2001 and 2006. They were written after the students first experienced shadowing the person doing the job that they would begin when they became doctors the August following their graduation. These reflective accounts are sometimes harrowing to read, often poignant and some are joyful; collectively they tell the current story of what it is like to begin work as a doctor in an NHS trust. We believe that through their reflections students have collectively given us a means to better understand some of the challenges faced in the NHS by patients and professionals alike.

The students' reflections were not originally intended for publication but were submitted as part of course work. However, we were determined to make these students' tremendous insights accessible to a wider readership and they gave their consent for us to do so. By publishing these accounts we invite both professionals and non-professionals to hear the students' perceptions of their initial experience of working within the NHS. By understanding and then addressing the issues students raise, we can ensure that our competent students become competent practitioners. It is the continuing memory of these experiences as told by the enthusiastic, bright and gifted undergraduate medical students who are the doctors of the future that helps us to remain involved in working to improve medical education – especially when the going gets tough.

The students' reflections offer a unique approach to understanding the enduring question of why new doctors sometimes struggle as they begin their first jobs. As students making the transition from medical school to hospital practice, they must cope with the reality of what it means for them to put their academic work into practice in the very human sphere of medicine. We hope that their work will inform curriculum development in the longer term. We are also convinced that their observations will help both service providers and patients to more fully understand some of the tensions that are inherent within the present healthcare system.

Kathy Feest
Karen Forbes
September 2006

About the authors

Kathy Feest is currently the Associate Dean and Director of the Foundation School in the Postgraduate Deanery, Severn Institute in Bristol. She is also a Special Advisor to Foundation Programmes for Modernising Medical Careers (MMC) in London. She grew up in America and began her career there in the theatre. She has worked in medical education in England for the past 25 years in many varying capacities.

Her first degree was in Social Anthropology. As the founding partner of a video production company she wrote and produced award-winning videos for both patients and professionals. She then went on to work as a Special Lecturer in Medical Education at the University of Bristol. She completed her PhD in Medical Education in 2003, which focused on the early experiences of junior doctors, and has since produced and written training courses for junior doctors. Kathy remains committed to working on behalf of junior doctors and as Director of the Foundation School continues to support the Shadowing course at the University of Bristol Medical School.

Karen Forbes is Consultant and Macmillan Professorial Teaching Fellow in Palliative Medicine at the United Bristol Healthcare Trust and the University of Bristol. She is the clinical lead for the Preparing for Professional Practice (Shadowing) course, course organiser for the fifth year oncology and palliative medicine teaching and course director for the MSc in Palliative Medicine at the University of Bristol. She also sits on the Standing Advisory Committee in Palliative Medicine of the Joint Committee for Higher Medical Training at the Royal College of Physicians and is thus involved in medical education and training at a national level. Her personal research interests are around how students are best prepared for dealing with death and dying.

List of contributors

Keith Amarakone
Caroline Ardron
Jemma Austin
Naomi Bacon
Lesley Bell
Rahul Bhatnagar
Anna Bibby
Zoe Brown
David Bruce
Tom Cant
Duncan Chambler
Hlupekile Chiipeta
Helen Daniel
Amy Davies
Emma Davies
Alison Drover
Stephanie Eckoldt
Helen Edwards
Hayley Evans
Ruth Evans
John Ferguson
Nikki Freeman
Laura Gosling
Warren Grant
Hugh Grant Peterkin
Emma Gray
Julia Gregg
Ben Grimshaw
Sameer Gujral
Rachael Hardaker
Kirstine Haslehurst
Lucy Hayden
Emily Henderson
Anna Hiller
Darren Hiller

Claire Hodgkinson
Jonathan Horsnell
Paul James
Preeti Khera
Catherine Kingscombe
Nadia Lewis
Andrew Lyon
Sabira Makati
Rebecca Mason
Maaike Moller
Joanne Morris
James Mottram
Kevin Ng
Dan Nguyen
Amy Nicol
Claire Novorol
Ellen Oakhill
Jenny Offord
Katherine Pennison
Elizabeth Pettitt
Angela Puffett
Tim Rattay
Louise Remedios
Sandeep Shetty
Ingrid Slade
Emma Smith
Charlotte Stagg
Claire Taylor
Sally Taylor
Rhys Thomas
Kathryn Westby
Polly Weston
Anne Whitehouse
Christopher Wilkins

Acknowledgements

This book is the culmination of work stretching back over seven years and incorporates many stories along the way. Inevitably there are many people who touched the process and without whose help this book would not have been published. We are grateful to you all.

We would like to thank first and foremost the students who have generously allowed us to share their stories with you. Without their overwhelmingly positive interest and caring about all aspects of their chosen profession there would be no story to tell. The other group of people that is ever present in these stories is patients. They are there on every page, but for the purposes of this book have necessarily remained anonymous. The pre-registration house officers (PRHOs) or Foundation Programme (F1) doctors and their senior medical colleagues, along with the nurses and the rest of the NHS trust teams, have also been crucial to these stories from the trusts and we thank them.

At Bristol University we would like to thank the original Steering Project Board and especially Dr Clive Roberts, Clinical Dean; Dr David Mumford, Director of Medical Education; and Dr Peter Fletcher as Chair. Very warm thanks to Professor Debbie Sharp who orchestrated the original bid and has constantly and tirelessly contributed to and championed the cause of medical education. Developing the original shadowing curriculum would not have been possible without the contribution of Gay Wood. Her many years in education were invaluable to us. We are also grateful to Professor Gareth Williams, Dean of the Faculty of Medicine and Dentistry at the University of Bristol, for supporting this project and encouraging us to bring these accounts into the public domain.

Kathy would like to thank the members of the ASME (Association for the Study of Medical Education) Educational Leadership course 2005 for their encouragement and especially Professor Steve Field for never doubting that these accounts could become a book and introducing her to Gillian Nineham at Radcliffe who agreed! The Severn Institute team have been unstinting in their constant support. Thanks especially to Clare Moorcroft. Jeannette Patterson, who has typed and retyped as well as chased trainees through several moves to ask permission to use their accounts, deserves a medal. Professor Davinder Sandhu, the Postgraduate Dean at the Severn Institute, has wholeheartedly supported and encouraged this work. And finally for Kathy there is the person who listens and reassures when no words will come and the deadline looms, and who remains central to her story and her life. Thank you Professor Terry Feest.

Karen would like to especially thank all of her colleagues in the Department of Palliative Medicine at the United Bristol Healthcare Trust and the University of Bristol who are always supportive of her work, but particularly Professor Geoff Hanks, for his continuous encouragement and mentorship, and, of course, her ever-loyal and patient family.

Both Kathy and Karen also owe a huge debt of gratitude to Professor Tim Bond, from the Graduate School of Education at the University of Bristol, who encouraged and nurtured their interest in narrative and without whose influence this book might never have been written.

To the many angels who have supported us as we have taken this journey. They know who they are.

Introduction

Reading a collection of reflective writing from medical students about a particular experience can teach us a great deal. We can learn what it is that students strive to learn. We can glimpse what it is they grapple with as they contemplate beginning to work within National Health Service (NHS) hospitals instead of 'just' learning in them. In their reflections, the powerful stories that they tell reveal what they consider they still need to know in order to practise and grow as professionals, as doctors and as people. This situates the work in a professional context. Additionally, through their collective eyes we are able to see a snapshot of what current hospital experience is like for them which is also meaningful to all of us, medical educators and lay people alike.

The reason this is so, according to anthropologists, is because medicine is an exquisitely perceptive indicator of the essential cultural characteristics of any period. Every culture develops a system of medicine which reflects its relationship to its general world view. The behaviour of individuals and groups when confronted by the intimidation, fear and dread of illness is inseparable from the notion that they have of themselves and is deeply embedded in the culture's general history.

When students share their revelations about the people they work with, and the situations they find themselves in, the world of the hospital is illuminated from their collective perspective. Their honesty and exuberance as well as, at times, their moral outrage are evident and powerful and provide insights into the current cultural climate we all live in.

Students' reflective writing is more than 'just' a personal expression of how a series of events unfolds. It is a means of exploring their professional experience. Gillie Bolton is convincing when she concludes that:

> political and social structures are increasingly hemming professionals in. Their right to make personal and moral judgments is being eroded everyday; they are being reduced to technicians, their skills to mere technical competencies. In order to retain political and social awareness and activity professional development work needs to be rooted in the public and political as well as in the private and personal.[1]

This book extends the personal and private nature of reflective accounts to the political and social. The personal becomes the political in professional groups. It is important that the voice of the personal is accounted for in the quest to improve the medical student's transition into professional practice.

The most important part of this book has been written by final year students from the University of Bristol. Their work forms the body of this book. Some readers may wish to go straight to the reflective accounts. Others may wish to learn more about the project that generated this work and this will be discussed below. If you are a professional turning straight to the reflections our hope is that you will be able to step aside from your professional socialisation and let the student accounts speak directly to you. We believe they offer a powerful and important view of our current complex medical system.

Background

The reflective accounts appearing in this book were originally written by students as part of an assignment during a Shadowing course that began at Bristol University in the spring of 2000. Educational reforms influenced by the General Medical Council (GMC) were enabling positive curriculum changes to take place throughout the country's medical schools.

The GMC is responsible for setting and monitoring the standards and outcomes for medical education in the UK both at undergraduate level and the first year of medical training after graduation. The GMC recognised the need to refocus medical school curricula, and in 1997 set out the requirements for the final year of medical education in the document *Tomorrow's Doctors*. The GMC wished to ensure that students were adequately prepared during their final year at medical school to begin work in NHS trusts. The GMC said:

> The broad aim must be to promote the development of a curriculum which corrects the existing faults of overload and didacticism. It must provide the graduate with the capacity and the incentive to acquire and apply new knowledge and with the ability to adapt to changing circumstances, many as yet unforeseen. There must also be a more focused short term aim; to equip the new graduate with the necessary knowledge, skills and attitudes to enable him or her to enter the pre-registration period of training with confidence and enthusiasm.[2]

The Chief Medical Officer responded to this challenge and commissioned half a dozen national curriculum development projects to encourage the creation of explicit collaboration between NHS organisations and medical schools. The projects were intended to ensure that what students were taught at medical school met the practical needs of the NHS. Bristol University's application was successful with its project entitled 'From Student to Doctor – Medical School to NHS Employment'; consequently the Shadowing course became one of the outcomes of these new developments in medical education.

The original research that underpinned the Shadowing course was developed over a year. The project board included a chief executive of an NHS trust, clinical tutors and other trust employees as well as representatives from the regional health authority and the university. The research using participant observation methodology was carried out in four of the region's NHS trust hospitals. Eight house officers were 'shadowed' for a week each, including their on-take and on-call experiences as well as their routine daily duties. In addition to this research 45 interviews were conducted within the trust. The primary outcomes of the research led the project board to develop the concept that fifth year undergraduates would 'shadow' the post that they would take up in August in order to familiarise them with their roles and responsibilities and enable them to make a smoother transition from student to doctor. The Shadowing course was thus developed as a two-week mandatory module within the university.

The detailed research identified five broad areas to include within the shadowing strand of the curriculum. They are:

- communication skills
- clinical administrative procedures
- roles and responsibilities

- clinical skills
- organisational skills.

The Shadowing course was subsequently designed and included the themes identified by the research. The course is monitored year on year and is consistently rated highly by the students and trainees.

Why ask medical students to write reflective accounts?

The Shadowing course is delivered over a two-week period. Students attend several workshops at the university and in the trusts, but the strength of the course is that the majority of it occurs in practice on the wards. Students shadow the first post they will begin in August following their successful graduation. The underlying principle of this element of shadowing was to introduce the students as 'nearly professionals' who would be joining their teams or communities of practice when they began working the following August. The course occurs before the Easter break and well before final exams.

The course was specifically designed to introduce students to aspects of their professional lives they would meet when they began their medical career. As 'life-long learning' or 'continuing medical education' would become important elements of their professional lives we determined that introducing these elements during a course which was based almost entirely 'in practice' was sensible.

Before the students began their shadowing in the trusts we explained that they would need to write a 'reflective account' of between 800 and 1,000 words about the experience. An audible groan usually filled the lecture theatre when this assignment was described. These were young medical students about to gain experience of their first jobs; they wanted to get on with it unhindered by anything as unusual as writing about and sharing that experience. They were asked to focus on the course themes as a point of departure but we explained why it was also important that they reflect on their experiences. In addition, we decided to offer prizes for the 'best' three reflective accounts.

As educationalists we were influenced by Donald Schön's work, which has become a part of the language of education. His notion of 'learning societies' seems particularly apt when viewed from the medical educator's perspective. All medical encounters are potential learning experiences within the medical learning society. How one becomes a life-long learner within this 'learning society' of professionals is the important question.[3,4]

One of Schön's major contributions was to bring the notion of 'reflection' into the core of understanding that explains what it is that professionals do. These ideas are particularly interesting to medical educationalists because much of medical education occurs in practice. 'Thinking on our feet' sums up the notion of reflection *in* action (or in practice) which, coupled with reflection *on* action (or practice), enables learners to situate their knowledge and learning and develop professional contexts that they can then draw upon.

In order to become 'reflective practitioners' professionals need to reflect on their experiences in practice. Both thinking on their feet in practice and thinking after the encounter about practice are invaluable to the learner. Writing about these experiences is a way of reframing and rethinking these experiences, which often leads to deeper levels of understanding and learning.

The students' accounts offer us the sorts of frames of reference that students develop as they come to terms with what they meet in the realities of their practice in the place where they will begin their careers. They offer us indications of what they discover on entering practice and the ways in which young trainees cope with their newly acquired professionalism.

How did we choose the accounts to publish?

Each year a group of medical educators read the reflective accounts, selecting the outstanding accounts to be put forward for the annual prizes. We were all consistently struck by how valuable these accounts were to the students. During the five years of the course we received nearly 900 accounts. The authors reread all of these accounts and shortlisted a third of them while noticing the recurring themes that emerged. These were then grouped under four main themes: 'General reflections', 'Relationships', 'Working within the system' and 'Death'. During the second reading of the shortlisted accounts we identified those that especially illuminated these themes and included the accounts that were particularly well written or said something in an especially meaningful or powerful way.

We then read all of the shortlisted 300 accounts again and chose the final accounts that appear here. At this stage we had not identified the previously shortlisted prize-winning accounts. When we did compare the accounts it was interesting to see that we had included most of those that had been either shortlisted or were prize winners. This triangulation of our work gives us a sense that we chose the 'right' accounts to publish. This does not mean that the students' work that does not appear is not valuable or important or in any way 'wrong'. Editing such personal and excellent work means making tough choices. The same powerful messages are in evidence in many of the accounts; however, some people express their sentiments more effectively than others. The messages conveyed in the choices we have made are indicative of the entire collection. We are convinced that students learned more from the exercise than either they or we had anticipated.

We have asked all of the students whose work appears here for permission to publish their accounts. All names and locations have been changed. To preserve anonymity we have included an alphabetical list of contributors. As this work belongs to students as they embark on their professional careers, we have decided that a proportion of proceeds from the sale of this book will be placed in a fund for Foundation Programme doctors. It is envisaged that we will set up a regional award for Foundation doctors.

The cast of characters

The people who appear in this book are all anonymous or their names have been changed, but they are also all real. In reading these accounts we need to remember that patients can be bewildered, frightened or threatened in the face of illness and disease and their confusion and pain is sometimes expressed as indignance, ingratitude or worse.

Neither patients nor professionals are immune to the emotional turbulence that we meet in illness. We are all, at some times in our lives, patients, and we expect doctors and other healthcare professionals to deal both with our situation and their own in an exemplary fashion. However, these accounts show all too clearly that all of these people are real; no one is perfect. This is to be expected in an honest portrayal of the delivery of healthcare.

These accounts are presented 'warts and all'. The accounts have been anonymised and edited for spelling and punctuation, but are otherwise presented as the students submitted them. The events described all occurred within NHS trust hospitals. Some of these accounts relate stories about staff that are not always flattering. In addition, they sometimes describe patients as difficult or demanding. Invariably, the patients described here are experiencing some of the most vulnerable moments of their lives. Both groups, patients and professionals, are dealing with extreme human experiences. These accounts privilege us to witness a range of human emotions that are sometimes difficult, but ultimately enlightening, to observe.

The shape of the book

Stories define us. They are the powerful medium we use to transfer information between ourselves. We tell each other about our day by telling a story including all the pertinent events of the day. In doing so, we recreate the experience for ourselves and sharing perhaps enables us to see or hear another view. Sometimes we are reminded by our listener, often an audience of one, that there are more reasons to act in a particular way than we may first perceive. The process of story telling helps us to rethink and sometimes reconsider our positions. When writing 'reflections' about an experience this is precisely what we are doing. We are attempting to learn from our experience; to redefine the experience we have had and to learn from what we have witnessed. Writing stakes our claim in our world and brings clarity to the events we observe. The choices we make about what to write about and reflect on are the areas that touch, concern, amuse or baffle us. They are the issues we seek to learn from.

We have chosen to let the students' accounts form a collective story. There are brief introductions to the final three sections of the book, but this is only to remind readers that they are moving into a different themed section. We have not analysed these stories here, choosing instead to let them speak for themselves. The stories in this collection are all based on real incidents that occurred in the past five years. We share them with you and hope that they will touch you as much as they have touched us over that time. If you are a professional medical educator, our hope is that these accounts will influence you in your practice. We hope they will remind you of some of the important themes that prompted you to become a medical professional in the first place. For all of us we are reminded of a Horace statement from *Satires* which continues to be relevant to our times: 'Change the name and it's about you, that story.'[5] These are stories that we can all identify with. These are the Shadowing stories.

References

1. Bolton G. *Reflective Practice*. London: Sage; 2006. p. xvi.
2. General Medical Council. *Tomorrow's Doctors*. London: GMC; 1993. p. 6.
3. Schön DA. *The Reflective Practitioner; how professionals think in action*. London: Arena; 1983.
4. Schön DA. *The Reflective Turn: case studies in and on educational practice*. New York: Teachers Press, Columbia University; 1991.
5. Horace. *Satires*. Bk. 1, no. 1, lines 69–70. Cited in von Herder JG and Moore G. *Selected Writings on Aesthetics*. New Jersey: Princeton University Press; 2006. p.442.

General reflections

Who, me?

What is a shadow? A phenomenon of nature; merely the silhouette of a 'real' object? Or is it more? Can this projected image of responsibility be more than a fretful mime artist attempting to emulate each and every move of its more experienced master? During my experience shadowing it became clear that even as a transient member of the healthcare team it is possible to be more than just a shadow; it is possible to be yourself.

This rather grandiose opening statement is attempting to get to the bottom of why I believe the PRHO shadowing experience is so valuable for medical students. It suggests that the two-week attachment enables medical students to see beyond the usual anonymity associated with a life of clinical training. After a few days of returning to the same ward, to meet the same staff with whom we care for the same patients, I began to see a light at the end of the tunnel; that is I began to see a place in the picture for myself.

> 'Andy! How are you?'
> 'Andy … could you just pass me those notes … that's it, cheers.'
> 'Andy do you know where Dr H is? I'm sure she was here a second ago …'

Who? … Me? … For the first time I was tongue tied on the ward and it wasn't because I couldn't remember the *name* of something or other; it was because someone had remembered mine! It was a genuine shock to feel aspects of my personality come out into the open during time spent with other members of staff. More than anything this experience made me feel human. The confidence gained when surrounded by familiar faces is noticeable in all aspects of life and I believe this effect is just as (if not more) potent when attempting to become part of the ward team.

On day one of the attachment I had mixed feelings as I approached the foreboding entrance to the trust. Aware that I might make a lasting first impression my insecurities began to surface: would I look like an incompetent fool? Would my new consultant laugh me off the ward and into an office job before I even had time to take off my coat? It felt like the first day at school all over again. The familiar building had taken on a different persona from past occasions when the trust played host to our medical education. The stairs seemed steeper, the directional signs suddenly seemed of vital importance and faces passed in the corridors were studied closely lest the owner should be your new closest colleague. This feeling of being overwhelmed became a common theme for the rest of the first day.

The hype surrounding the attachment meant I had high expectations of day one. Shadowing had been described as a 'moment of educational clarity where our goals become clear'. Maybe a little dramatic but most ex-students I spoke to certainly found it to be the best insight into what the future held as a real doctor.

As it transpired it wasn't the epiphany I had imagined it would be. My new ward was a busy one and my arrival prompted the usual muffled hellos that herald the start of most of my clinical placements.

As the day wore on my house officer's job seemed to be an endless list of tasks I had no knowledge of whatsoever. As the day ended I doubted there would ever be a time when I was master of this role (with my very own shadow).

As the attachment unfolded and the feeling of acceptance I described earlier began to take effect I began to relax and take stock of my situation. I came to realise it was the simple things that were making the experience special. On one occasion a few days into my first week it fell to me to take some arterial blood. I'd tried and succeeded before in other hospitals but somehow this attempt would be special. This was to be my ward in the future and it felt so important to 'start as I meant to go on'. As it transpired my less than steady hand came good; I successfully acquired some arterial blood and left the ward that evening with a spring in my step. There were other small victories such as this; a correctly written discharge summary or the timely spare biro produced from nowhere for the busy consultant. Over the week the accumulation of events such as these made me realise the job is not one huge task to master in one, but a collection of smaller duties that are steadily achieved.

In conclusion it would seem that the hype was not totally unfounded. The shadowing attachment has given me a steely confidence that not only do I think I can do my job, but I might even bring a certain something of myself to it that others cannot. In the future, if someone asks me from the younger years how I found my shadowing I will be quick to praise the experience, even hype it if you will. However, I will be quick to add my own proviso; the experience will only be what they make of it. It requires us to make the most of our time with the established team to find our niche within it. By working hard to see the positives over the hurdles then even a lowly shadow can foresee a bright future.

Humdrum satisfaction

> Hospitals began as a casual ward for lepers and the like to die in, and they continued as places where medical students learned their art on the bodies of the poor.[1]

On the Thursday of shadowing week my surgical shadow-caster was on take. Late in the afternoon, while he was attending to some ward work, he was asked to go down to the Surgical Admissions Unit. He put down the phone, paused, tapped the desk pensively then told me to 'look into it'. Shorn from my shadow I set off, eyes a little sharper, heart a little faster.

Upon arrival at SAU I found a prim, composed lady seated expectantly, accompanied by four lightly packed bags. Once I was allocated a room I went through her history with her, and then examined her. As I expected from her history I found a painful irreducible right-sided inguinal hernia on examination (and an irregularly irregular pulse).[2] After consulting a senior house officer I took and sent off blood samples, requested an electrocardiogram and sited a cannula. All simple acts, and ones I have been trained to perform.

I picked this small incident because it encapsulates two important points I learned as a result of the added responsibility given to me during shadowing week. The first was related to my history and examination skills. I'd elicited and documented some slight depressive symptoms when discussing the lady's mood and well-being, but I didn't push the point when she brushed me off. It later transpired that she had an appointment to see a psychiatrist shortly, to look into a possible diagnosis of depression. The discovery did not affect her treatment, but it taught me that (gently) asking an extra question can reveal much; a history is not a proforma.

I've been told examining a patient is like a 'game' or 'a dance'. I've been told to treat the whole process in the same way I would a driving test. That advice might be sound for finals, but, in the acute clinical setting, it quickly becomes clear that while examining may well be an art, it has no artifice. When I watched the surgical registrar examine the lady's hernia I recognised that I was an amateur. He palpated her hernia with a firmer and far more accomplished hand. I had been a little hesitant for fear of causing pain. Years of experience separated us.

The second 'learning point' came to me the next day when I was talking to the patient on the ward after her operation. In the course of our chat she joked about the fiddliness of her undergarments and how I should get married 'quick sharp'. It was then I realised that the day before I'd acquired something of a 'hunt the pathology' attitude that diminished both the patient and myself. This attitude can result in the mentality that Foucault so despised; that is, a student so alienated from her/his activities that 'what the student sees is not the atlas as a representation of the body but the body as a representation of the atlas'.[3] Instead of this, effort has to be expended to maintain the humanity and dignity of all involved in the medical world. So, if I do my job well and stay attentive to all around me I can go home agreeing with the poet and doctor William Carlos Williams when he said 'it's the humdrum, day-in, day-out, everyday work that is the real satisfaction of the practice of medicine'.[4]

The attitude of quiet attentive caring excellence that I have witnessed in the doctors I admire most is the greatest learning experience I'll ever have. I have known this before but, as with all truths, each iteration brings further light and clarity. In this respect shadowing week gave me a sliver of an insight into how I might become, in my own way, like the doctors I've learned most from.

On a more pragmatic note, one of the most important things the PRHO I shadowed taught me was that scrupulous time (and note) keeping made the job less stressful, the ward more efficient and better served the patients. He prioritised easily and accurately so that the macro-organism of the ward moved more smoothly for his presence. Investigation ordering, form filling and drug chart adjusting are all skills I am yet to be proficient in. I perform them with the slow awkward concentration of a middle-aged man being taught to knit. But, though clunky at first, with practice he can move through the wool precisely and swiftly, just as I hope to move through the administrative side of my future job.

What else have I learned? I've learned what a woman looks like when she is told that her husband died in a nursing home while she was in hospital, away from him for the first time in 15 years. I've also learned how to hold someone's hand as they cry through the realisation that their tummy-ache has turned into a large bowel excision, a hysterectomy and a probable diagnosis of cancer. I've learned I have a long way to go, a huge amount to learn, and that 'if the physician attends only to disease and ignores suffering, he may cure but he fails to heal'.[5]

Oh, I've also learned (again) that often the best route out of any problem is letting everyone talk until it's gone. And not taking yourself too seriously (I don't normally spout Foucault) is critical to maintaining good working relationships.

The learning skills I've identified I need to develop in my F1 year? I know them and they are many: I'm competent at blood taking, less competent at catheter insertion and so on. These things will, I hope, come with time. My history and examination skills (of paramount importance) also need time. I feel more than ever that in order to prove Orwell wrong and progress I require a rigorous and holistic awareness of myself, my colleagues and, most importantly, my patients …

Notes

1. Orwell G. *Decline of the English Murder and Other Essays*. London: Penguin with Secker and Warburg; 1965. p. 43.
2. There was a part of me that was pleased at the finding! … There is a definite 'buzz' to be had from finding a sign that has not previously been noted (especially as a junior). But the 'buzz' is not a wholly appropriate response; surely it is somewhat callous?
3. Armstrong D. *The Political Anatomy of the Body*. Cambridge: Cambridge University Press; 1983. p. 2.
4. Williams W. *The Autobiography*. New York: New Directions; 1967.
5. Brody H. *The Healer's Power*. Yale: Yale University Press; 1993.

Shadowy reflections on shadowing week

Full of joy at the prospect of my forthcoming job at the highly regarded trust, I arrived on my first day of shadowing overflowing with enthusiasm, random medical knowledge and free drug-representative tourniquets. Such was my keenness to embark on my imminent career that my fervour was only mildly dented when I found out that my predecessor on the ward and revered leader for the week was away on holiday. However, knowing that flexibility is a key skill for junior doctors in the modern NHS, I overcame my disappointment and, using all my powers of lateral thinking and ingenuity, decided to shadow the covering house officer instead. Unfortunately he had rather selfishly chosen the previous day to get married and thought that this warranted a day off work, so he too was unable to be the shining example of good medical practice that I was searching for. Gusto seeped out of me like fluid around a badly placed venflon as, with my head hanging, I decided to leave the hospital and shelve my aspirations of medical greatness for another day. It was in this slightly dented and rather vulnerable state that I ran into the team I would be working for during the second part of my job, who were about to embark on a respiratory ward round. Their careless talk of BIPAP and chest drains renewed my energy, and I cheerily assumed my appropriate position in ward round formation (behind the house officer, in front of the third year students) as we bounced off to the next ward.

Five hours later I was mentally listing the other options available to an intelligent Bristol graduate with incomplete medical training and science A levels, and by the time we finally finished at 7 o'clock at night I was internally cursing the naïve and foolish girl who had started the day with such buoyancy. That evening's reflections on my first day were of a dark and murky nature, and the fortnight of shadowing looked set to be as dim as the name implied. Fortunately, however, the proceeding day emphasised the chiaroscuro of life (and medicine) by dawning bright and clear, meteorologically and metaphorically. By 9 o'clock, having completed two surgical ward rounds, discharged three patients and had time for a congratulatory cup of coffee, I was beginning to see the bigger picture. Three cheers for surgery: clearly it was here that quality of life (such as is available to a PRHO) was to be found.

The week continued in this sunny tranquil fashion, leaving my house officer and me plenty of time for leisurely tours of radiology and illuminating conversations with pharmacists. Equally, opportunities to implement clinical skills arose regularly, and I gaily seized each one, taking advantage of the pressure-free environment to consolidate my slightly vague abilities to the effect that at the end of the shadowing course I felt fully equipped to take blood, catheterise and cannulate in any situation. Although obviously to do so in *any* situation may be inappropriate. I even drained a seroma one day.

Unfortunately there was one incident that occurred which may have de-skilled me for life by creating a mental aversion to the procuring of arterial blood gases. The experience did teach me a valuable lesson, however, about clinical skills, communication skills and the need to appreciate the patient in context so, on balance, perhaps it was a worthwhile trade.

The patient in question was a 60-year-old lady who had just undergone a bilateral mastectomy for breast carcinomas. Post-operatively her sodium had dropped to 117 causing her to fit overnight and to experience hypotensive episodes while off the ward, resulting in mild panic for the nurses with her, and her swift return to the ward before any investigations could be completed. Regular monitoring of her sodium was encumbered by her minimal veins and the desire to avoid using a tourniquet on her arms to minimise the risk of lymphoedema. Following my house officer's advice that a femoral stab was the only technique likely to yield any of the red stuff, I aimed for her groin on the sole occasion I was to attempt to take her blood. Initially she was stoical about the needle digging deep into her flesh, and it was only after approximately 20 minutes that she began first to moan slightly and then to cry. I have not been the cause of someone else's tears since I was at playschool, and never a fully grown woman of my mother's generation. I felt awful.

As I sat on her bed holding her hand she told me how much it all hurt, and how she was *just so tired*. I realised that in the past 24 hours she had lost both her breasts, experienced her first ever fit and come very close to death. More potently perhaps was the release from fear, now her cancer had been removed, mixed with trepidation about the histology results. In her situation I'd be more than exhausted; I'd be terrified, and traumatised by the way my body had decided to betray me. The medical intervention I was receiving, rather than reassuring me, would scare me even further. The pain of repeated blood tests was a trigger for all this emotion rather than the cause (or so I told myself), and this made me realise the reality of hospital admissions for many patients; doctors who spend their whole lives inside hospitals, and see a variety of patients daily, can fail to appreciate that for the patient this is probably the most stressful and scary thing they have ever experienced. I hope this is something I will never forget as a doctor.

As well as appreciating the importance of empathy and taking time to listen, this episode also made me aware that my femoral stab technique would have to be improved upon dramatically if I were to survive my house-officer year without reducing every patient to tears. Another invaluable lesson learned. In fact I found the whole shadowing period to be suffused with similar learning points, from trivial things like knowing where to put completed blood forms, to seminal revelations about the nature of my own approach to patients and the tendency and validity of trying to keep messy, time-consuming emotions at bay. All of this will affect my clinical practice for the better next year, assuming, that is, that I manage to fit in some revision for finals around my new found, super-empathic, understanding approach to life.

Shades of the future: an account of what is to be my first house job

Day one

The corridors of the trust are grimily familiar as I stride sweating from the humid morning rain into the Postgraduate Centre. The time is 7.55. For a brief second the acrid smell of the men's toilets jars in my nostrils: a classic NHS welcome. I say a cheery hello to a distant professor; he smiles kindly, but looks a little surprised. 'Why shouldn't he?' I think to myself. After all it is early, and while he is large and significant in my small world there can be no doubt that in his much larger world, I almost don't exist at all. If anything, I am an arm in a lecture theatre, an untucked shirt on a ward round or perhaps an irritating shadow cast across the operating table. Not for long, I tell myself, soon I'll be significant, not important perhaps, but useful; no longer in the way, no longer an unwanted irritation, no longer a STUDENT.

The old common room flashes past as I rush deeper into the hospital. I spare a split second of nostalgia for the pool table but I know I won't be going there today. No indeed! For today I have more important work to do – I am to be shadowing what will be my first ever real job. I am excited, I feel a whiff of reality in the air. Will I be able to cope? Will the SHO like me? Will I like him? Will the nurses crucify me? What is my consultant like? Will ANY of the patients believe that the wide-eyed, pasty-faced student before them is to be their doctor in less than four months?

I walk onto the ward. It is 8 am. There is a male nurse looking important in the office. Dark blue uniform, pursed lips and half-moon spectacles. I introduce myself with what I judge to be the correct amount of enthusiasm/deference. His mouth proclaims pleasure to meet me; his eyes are not quite sure if they agree. The only other person in the office is a girl in the corner reading a book; she doesn't look up, and I feel a little shy so I don't introduce myself. I indulge in a light breakfast of ward Quality Street. (There is only toffee left and I feel acid squirt as it plops into my stomach.)

James, the PRHO currently at the helm of the joyful thingumology house job that is to be mine, arrives on the ward. I met him the day before at orientation so I feel a little light banter is in order. He is wearing a black shirt, so I ask him merrily if this is a reflection of extreme right political leanings. We have a bit of a laugh. Next, the SHO walks in and is even more frank in his response to the shirt. 'Nice outfit, James; you look like a Nazi.' He sits down at the computer. Finally, the registrar arrives and taking one look at his PRHO ejaculates, 'Right then Sturmbahnfuhrer, shall we do the ward round?', and looking at the girl in the corner, 'Hello, who are you?' 'Good morning doctor, I am Helga, a medical student from Germany, visiting on elective.'

Inside my head someone is dragging their nails down a blackboard.

Day two

Well, after that inauspicious start, the rest of the day went fine. I took notes on the ward round, learned about the computer, hunted for some missing x-rays, sorted out a few patients' drug charts, wrote a few TTAs and it didn't even seem all that hard. This morning has been pretty much the same and still no one thinks I am a fraud. It is 10.30 and everyone is having coffee and toast in the mess and talking about how irritating being bleeped for such and such a job is. The PRHO is watching MTV and muttering something enthusiastic about Gwen Stefani dressed as a pirate. The mess is 'awesome' I have decided – free toast, great sofas and Sky TV. I don't even miss the pool table. This whole job in fact seems pretty easy … I can't see what all the fuss is about. My PRHO looks at me and, as if reading the over-confidence in my mind, says, 'We are on take tonight, mate, so I'd eat something now so you don't get too hungry later …'. As it isn't even lunchtime that sounds pretty ominous. The bleep goes. James reads me the number and I answer it. It's the clinic nurse from down the hall. James is wanted to help in pre-op assessment.

'Here we go,' says James and he springs off the sofa. I gulp coffee and follow him out the door like a flurry of leaves in the wake of a speeding car. As we walk towards pre-op assessment, the bleep goes again. We pop into x-ray and James uses the phone. It's a GP admission. Abdo pain, query mesenteric artery ischaemia. 'Well, I'm not going to argue with that,' he says, looking impressed. We ring the bed manager and write down the patient's details so we remember to see him later, then it is back on course for pre-op. The first patient comes in; we run through all the questions. It's all going well, they seem to be safe for an anaesthetic, then suddenly the patient's shirt is off and I am listening to the heart and rather than a reassuring lub dub, lub dub, I hear a less than reassuring lub shhh, lub shhh. 'I think this person has a murmur, James.' 'Oh really?' He listens in as well. 'They certainly do,' he agrees, 'but what we do about that I am not sure. We had better go and ask someone.' We wander out looking for an SHO. There isn't one but one of the brainier-looking PRHOs is standing around for some reason. We describe the situation to him and he starts burbling something intellectual about cardiovascular criteria and anaesthetics … I see James switch off just as readily as his colleague commences showing off. Just then the clinic nurse appears, looking stressed. 'What are you doing chatting? We've got a massive backlog of people waiting out there. The consultant is on holiday, I've got the flu … nag, nag, naggety nag. BEEP BEEP BEEP. There goes the bleep again. Suddenly, everything seems very stressful indeed.

James looks coolly down at the plastic box on his belt. He ignores the nurse, and looks at me: 'You take this call; I'll phone anaesthetics to find out about the man with the murmur and then I'll see whether my SHO will cover the pre-op clinic for me.' I take a second, and then ring the number I have just been given. It's Sister upstairs on SAU: a patient has just arrived from A&E in great pain. They're writhing around on their bed, they're screaming, it might be appendicitis, they need analgesia now, could you get James to come up here immediately, it is really very urgent.

Responsibility and rewards

The morning in pre-op pretty much set the tone for that whole day and to some extent the rest of the week. We ran from ward to ward, clerking new patients, sorting out the problems of established patients and generally working hard. I realised that my job was not in fact going to be dominated by eating toast and watching Gwen Stefani on television in the mess. In actual fact looking after patients and doing the jobs that their required management created was (surprise, surprise) the main event. After a few more days of doing this I began to realise that although much of what I was seeing was familiar – after all, I have been in and out of hospitals for four years as a medical student – there was something really very different about actually being in the front line. The immediacy of problems struck me; the dependence of other staff on oneself was suddenly apparent; the reality of patients' suffering and their need for reassurance, explanations and support became clearer than it ever had been before. I realised that as a medical student you are somehow distanced from problems that at first glance look as if they are right in front of you. It is almost as if there is a pane of smoked glass between you and the person in the bed. Your powerlessness saves you from the reality of their situation; because you can't do anything, you don't have to think about it or take any responsibility for it. When you are a junior doctor suddenly that pane of glass is removed. This is exhausting, for in a flash every job has to be done: other people will experience consequences if YOUR tasks are not completed. The good old days of being able to put off work till tomorrow are over. Fortunately, however, if the reality of people's problems is more real so too is the reward to be had from sorting them out. Heading home at 9 pm after a hard day of providing real care for real people is a lot more gratifying than sloping off at lunchtime on a Tuesday having made up some bullshit about playing mixed lacrosse.

The end

There are lots of other things I would love to talk about: difficulties surrounding shoe politics in the men's changing rooms in theatre, the delights of shadowing the nurses, and an embarrassing moment involving an anal abscess. However, this is meant to be quite a short piece of work and a lot of the other things I would like to say can probably wait. If the essay seems a little unfinished then perhaps that is because subconsciously I feel that way about the shadowing. It's not a complete story; it's an introduction. It may not be entirely satisfying; but it's a welcome indication of exciting things to come.

Human elements of the job strike home

You've got wires, going in
You've got wires, coming out of your skin
You've got tears, making tracks
I've got tears that are scared of the facts.

You've got wires, going in,
You've got wires, coming out of your skin.
There's dry blood, on your wrist

Your dry blood, on my fingertip.
(Athlete, 'Wires', from the album *Tourist*)

'Arterial line … CVP … GCS of 6 … intropes … Schwann-Ganz … 'trace' … PEEP … CPAP … central line …'

Having spent six years as a medical student absorbing and accumulating the weird and wonderful language and culture that is 'medicine', the intensive care unit heralds a plethora of undiscovered terminology, procedures and emotions. This intimidating and alien environment houses the sickest patients in the hospital and, as such, is predominantly the domain of experienced physicians and incredibly talented nursing staff.

As a medical student (and soon-to-be F1 doctor), the opportunity to observe these unique creatures in their natural habitat was somewhat humbling. In the vast majority of cases, the ability to implement knowledge and maintain respect for patients and relatives while communicating effectively with other team members was extremely impressive.

When applying for the rotation incorporating 'peri-op', the term 'supernumerary' seemed a little ambiguous. Secretly, did it imply 'not-really-needed'? The shadowing experience emphatically eliminated this fear; despite occupying an unquestionably 'junior' role, the PRHO in peri-op medicine can contribute fully and invaluably to the combined multidisciplinary team. Given the emotionally demanding aspects of working with very ill patients, and the unique, almost intimate setting of ITU, the interprofessional relationships are of paramount importance. The opportunity to meet members of the medical and nursing teams as a student relieves a degree of trepidation prior to starting the job in August. At a time when nerves will undoubtedly be prominent, a familiar face will be an extremely welcome feature of day one!

In reality, it is arguable that a 'supernumerary' position actually affords the relative luxury of providing compassionate, empathic care without the all-too-familiar restriction of time. The setting of ITU seems an apt environment in which to provide both patients and relatives with this resource; namely a doctor willing to prioritise the non-medical aspect of patient care. While far from intentional, it is indisputable that time restraints impair the ability of a busy doctor to exercise the full range of their empathic and communication skills. Following consultation with past and present PRHOs, common frustrations frequently arise:

> It feels like all those communication skills sessions were a waste of time. Taking time to just talk to patients or relatives has become a luxury I can't afford. Sending off blood forms, spending hours running up and down six flights of stairs to charm the radiology receptionist, trying to decipher the computer system … I barely have time for a coffee and a loo break, never mind spending an hour with relatives who really do need to talk. (Anon PRHO)

This sentiment was echoed by colleagues shadowing medical and surgical house officers at many hospitals. Hence my feeling of privilege while shadowing a job where my PRHO was largely free from such frustrations. A striking example of this was one particularly memorable experience during the job shadowing fortnight. A 58-year-old lady was transferred to the intensive care unit with worsening respiratory failure, connected to seemingly innumerable tubes, wires and medical paraphernalia, echoing the poignant lyrics of a current popular song (see above).

At a relatively young age, the devastation of this lady's children, contemplating the unexpectedly premature loss of their mother, was overwhelming. Having had little experience with dying patients or grieving relatives, I worried that any word I could offer would be woefully inadequate. However, observing my PRHO communicate with the relatives reassured me that even simple measures may provide significant support. Her combination of clear, simple medical explanations (when requested), empathic expressions of support and respectful maintenance of distance ensured the relatives felt welcomed into, and not threatened by, the ITU setting.

Prior to the shadowing course, the primary aims of most fifth year students were to familiarise ourselves with the potentially 'mundane' aspects of the job. Admittedly, we were all obsessed with the seemingly endless and daunting administrative tasks:

> 'Which bloods go in which bottle?'
> 'How do I call the porters?'
> 'What am I actually supposed to write in the notes?'
> 'Where can I go for a quick cry when the consultant shouts at me on a ward round?'
> 'Where is the mess?'

Whilst all these fundamental questions (and more) were vital lessons from the shadowing course, in retrospect, the 'human' elements of the job were the truly striking learning points. Whether it be reassuring worried relatives, timely hand-holding with a terrified patient, or recognising when a mutually supportive debrief with colleagues is needed, this job will present a huge emotional learning curve. However, the shadowing fortnight dramatically reduces the daunting prospect of beginning this new adventure, and even began to reassure me that I could actually be a good doctor quite soon …

I only hope I can have the same effect on my shadow a year from now!

This ugly duckling

Before

> 'Fantastic! Two weeks off revising and worrying about exams. Instead I'll be watching someone do some practical things. I can handle that, and might learn valuable finals tips too – after all, this is an "all access pass" to a PRHO who went through it all recently. I am looking forward to what I can get out of it.'

After

> 'I've always worked with short-term goals in mind; to get through the next block of exams. I've never realistically focused on the bigger picture of working as a doctor. It's never been so tangible before … until now. I'm thinking about the job I am preparing for, though I still don't fully comprehend what lies ahead. At least I am looking further

forward than I have before and I am glad for what shadowing has shown me.'

What happened in between

It's my responsibility

My life as a medical student has been spent making excuses:

> 'I'm only a third year, we haven't covered that yet!'
> 'I'm not sure about that, I'm just a fourth year medical student.'
> 'Well, since I'm in my fifth year, it's been so long since we did it, I don't remember!'

The first practical 'tip' given to me by the pre-registration house officer (PRHO) I was shadowing was to think before I did or signed anything:

> 'At the end of the day it's your responsibility. You have to make decisions and be able to justify them.'

Wondering what I would do in a given situation with no one to check up on me, it was not a lack of knowledge that was unsettling, but the thought of making a final commitment. This would be on paper, for all to see and there would be no scope for the short white coat and excuses that I had shielded myself with before. As a medical student I have *played* at being doctor, making guesses and deliberating about real-life decisions. I was safe in the knowledge that I did not have to take responsibility. Considering this raised several questions for me. Could I do this? What if I made a mistake? What if I did not know what to do?

With these thoughts in mind, as the days progressed, I found myself actively watching and thinking, instead of passively observing. I noticed that minute by minute the house officer was making decisions and taking actions for which they were responsible: requesting investigations, filling drug charts, prescribing fluids, organising ward rounds, admitting patients and booking theatre lists. To top it all off, this was done with a fluency I knew I did not possess, let alone feel able to conjure up in time for August. I looked on and wondered how the relative 'swan' before me could have once been an awkward 'ugly duckling', as I now felt.

As busy as you make it

Aside from taking responsibility, I noticed that the way in which the house officer carried out the job was individual. No one stipulated how to prioritise jobs, when to take a lunch break or when all the work was done (though nurses and seniors might ask for specific things). No two days were the same. This prospect fascinated me: job ownership. It dawned on me that this was not *a job*, to be done mindlessly over and over, unchanging and unyielding. But it would be *my* job to take pride in and to be done and learned from, as I felt, in the best possible way. To a degree the role was as busy as one made it and it was up to the individual to organise and streamline time. For example, going down to radiology to request an investigation, the house officer was asked for more clinical information and plain films. Unfortunately, this meant another trip back to base to pick them up and shuttle them back down again. Taking everything down together would save time and also impress on the radiologists that you were organised and meant business! I am looking forward to a job I can make my own.

Your time is valuable ... to others

A lady on the ward, a 40-year-old language teacher, was distraught. Having been in a road traffic accident, suffering bilateral leg fractures, she was in hospital await-ing an operation. Her husband and two young children lived two hours away and the date of her operation had been repeatedly cancelled. Low in mood and at the end of her emotional tolerance she broke down in floods of tears, saying she could bear waiting no longer, when the PRHO and I went to see her. She was obviously very distressed. The PRHO took her hand and, for 10 minutes, reassured her through tear-filled conversation. After some time, the patient dried her eyes and began to smile. She said she felt alone and that all day no one had come to speak with her. To have someone listen to her was enough to make a difference. No one else had offered their time to her that day except the house officer.

I want to be able to make that difference. It was something that did not require the knowledge of the obscure causes of hypokalaemia, but the sensitivity and awareness that another person would appreciate your time. For the first time in the shadowing week I felt that this was something I could do, and I would be proud to take responsibility for. I can make a difference.

The importance of trust

Being a shadow is an experience which I feel, on the whole, has been the largest part of medical school. I have learned over the past five years the art of blending in, following blindly and generally hanging around. Of being an apparition in a corner, an appendage listening to consultations, of existing, but what as, no one is quite sure.

Indeed, being a fifth year medical student is even more of a grey area than ever before. It's like being 'between stools', as my mother used to say, when I had reached a particularly troublesome or tiresome stage of my development. This was highlighted no more acutely than when shadowing. During this time I was still a student but I was also the person who, in four months time, would be part of the team. The person who would be at the end of the bleep, the person needed to do jobs, to look after patients, to pass the buck to, to ...

But I wasn't there yet, I wasn't a doctor, I hadn't crossed the finishing line. I didn't have the magic piece of paper or those special letters in front of my name which would, overnight, make me capable of doing everything that I am unable to do today. I was, and still am, just a shadow. Yet in order to be a doctor you need to practise just that, being a doctor, not being a shadow.

For those around me, in a world where hierarchy and definition mean every-thing, this was understandably difficult. It was surprising how different people responded to me in very different ways. There was the scared 'You're not qualified, you're not allowed to do that!' group. Then there was the 'Oh, it's all right, you're still a student, you don't need to do that' group. They were both well meaning enough; however, they both failed to realise that when it comes to the time when 'I have to do that', I won't be able to because they won't let me do it now.

Fortunately there were those who were more willing to trust, to let me practise being a doctor, and this I suppose defined for me what medicine is truly about: trust. To work as a team you need to be able to trust those around you and in return they need to be able to trust you. Those who trusted me were brave, because real trust takes time and, despite not knowing me well, they were willing to believe that I was up to the job and more importantly to believe that I was aware of my own limitations, that I was safe.

It therefore astonishes me the level of trust that patients place in us on a daily basis. How truly brave they are to literally place their lives in our hands. Trust, I realised, is not only a privilege but also a responsibility. I had a sense of not wanting to let my colleagues down, not to betray those who had trusted me and certainly not to betray the trust of those that I was caring for.

An 87-year-old lady was admitted with obstruction, which turned out to be a gastric volvulus. This was decompressed using conservative means and as result she felt a lot better. She was relieved because she was adamant that she was not going to have surgery. She had been in almost a year ago for an operation and had only just survived. She was older now and indeed frailer and felt that another operation would be the end of her. She was a bright and articulate lady who knew her own mind and had made her own decision. However, those around her did not agree and felt that she would benefit from a more permanent surgical solution. The surgeon was willing to operate and her daughters wanted what was best for their Mum. Between them they persuaded themselves and her to go for the op, to 'stop her suffering'. She wasn't convinced but she signed the consent forms nonetheless. She trusted us. Tragically she died less than 24 hours after surgery. I have never felt so angry or guilty about a patient, I felt that I had let her down, and I cried – lots.

I was on MAU and I had some wonderful people to support me. I clerked patients in, ordered tests and planned treatments, reporting back to the more senior doctors if I was unsure what to do and asking them to sign forms as necessary. I, along with all the other juniors, presented my patients to the consultants on the evening ward round. It was like being a doctor with stabilisers, a pseudo-doctor, and at the end of the two weeks I felt for the first time, 'Oh my God, maybe I really can do this'.

I was reminded of the moment when I was peddling away thinking that Dad still had a steadying hand on my back mud-guard, only to realise that he was standing 20 metres back beaming away in the proud paternal way that Dads do. I was wobbling lots, but I was doing it.

You don't need to know about working time directives or to fill in your handy white 'file-o-facts' to become a doctor. You simply need to be given the opportunity to get on with it. After all, that's what we are going to have to do in August, when we step out of our shadows and more importantly when 'Dr' instantly means trustworthy.

Keeping alcohol in check

I will describe and reflect upon an event that occurred during my 10 days of PRHO shadowing. In doing so I hope to understand myself better and to set 'learning needs' to aid in similar situations during my F1 year and subsequent career.

Monday

9.30 am	Arrived at the hospital to be greeted by the Foundation Programme Director.
9.35 am	Invited to join junior doctors on a night out. Informed that drinks will be free in the hospital social club.

9.50 am	PRHOs bleeped. Met consultant (who was on A&E surgical take). The consultant gave me his ward bleep should I need to be contacted. Spent the day clerking and presenting patients.
4.30 pm	Finished in the hospital. Sent home by consultant and told to return tomorrow afternoon (as it was never busy in the mornings). Spent the evening watching *Neighbours*, shopping in Sainsbury's and glancing over acute pancreatitis in *Oxford Handbook of Clinical Medicine*.
8 pm	Visited hospital social club with other medical students.
10 pm	Finished off my third free drink and grabbed a taxi to town with everyone else.
10.15 pm	Arrived at an infamous late night bar. Mess President gave each and every one of us a free toffee vodka, which is not a pleasant drink when spilt!
11 pm	Drinking games began: house doctors vs shadow doctors. We lost 2–1.
2 am	Taxi home via the local kebab shop.

Tuesday

8.30 am	Consultant's ward bleep woke me up. Simple message needed to be passed on to other vascular PRHO.
8.35 am	I realised I was very hungover, possibly still drunk.
12 pm	Felt slightly more normal. Attempted to speak to consultant. Failed due to expressive dysphasia. Told to go back to bed.
4.30 pm	Consultant bleeped me and asked if I wanted to see a patient or to call it a day. Having done nothing all day, I gratefully accepted the latter and returned to bed.

Wednesday

Still slightly dazed with a mild dysarthria, but no physical pain. Worked with consultant from 9 am to 5 pm in an attempt to make up for my poor effort on Tuesday.

Explanation of choice

This was considerably lazy and poor behaviour from me. It is possible as a student to get away with such behaviour as our responsibilities are few and far between but the 10 days of PRHO shadowing have made me realise that next year will be different.

It is said that a patient is an alcoholic only if they drink more than their doctor. Alcohol is, for right or wrong, closely linked with socialising within the UK and almost every form of employment promotes drinking alcohol to some extent, from manual labouring through to professional skilled work. This in itself may not be a bad thing as there are benefits to the occasional and light drink. Drinking in excess, either chronically or acutely (binge drinking), has, however, many detrimental effects, sometimes leading to events involving the health service and/or the police.

I will openly confess to drinking in excess in the past, and no doubt in the future too, but managing and being aware of my limits is vital. I chose to describe and discuss this event because I became deeply aware of the implications of being too hungover, or too drunk, to practise safely as a doctor. Reflecting on this event has highlighted some of the objectives of the PRHO Shadowing Programme.

- Knowledge, skills and attitudes: a certain attitude is required of doctors. This applies to medical students as well, but, as previously mentioned, the lower responsibilities allow this attitude to be bent or stretched while a student. I feel very strongly that being hungover, or actually drunk, is in complete conflict with this required attitude.
- Multidisciplinary team and the doctor's role: teamwork is central to working as a Foundation doctor. Working when hungover or drunk, or not turning up for work, all increase the burden on those working around you.
- Being a reflective practitioner: alcohol issues can become problems slowly over time. A 'reflective practitioner' will hopefully notice these issues before they become problems and act accordingly.

Self-reflection and awareness are extremely important in managing alcohol safely and with this in mind I have drawn up a personal plan to practise safely as a F1 doctor.

- Attitude: I intend to consider my behaviour when socialising, ensuring that I can function competently, safely and confidently when working.
- Teamwork: I intend to support my colleagues by maintaining a good level of work at all times and not allowing alcohol to decrease my abilities.
- Responsibility: if I should find myself unable to work safely then it is my responsibility to inform the correct people. This applies to both the morning after a single occasion, but also (through reflective practising) in the long term should help be needed. Furthermore, it is my responsibility to inform the correct people should I feel a colleague is unable to work safely.

Practically speaking, this leads to the following limitations.

- A *'teetotal'* night is one that requires me to drive, be responsible for others or work before a night's sleep.
- A *'light'* night is one that allows a night's sleep and precedes a day's work.
- A *'heavy'* night is one that has at least 24 hours before my next shift, allowing adequate recovery. I should take all reasonable effort to avoid driving during that 24-hour period.

Evaluation of this experience

In all honesty, I do not believe I have a drinking problem! Through this reflection I have taken a simple awareness of poor student behaviour and have drawn it out for serious consideration. I appreciate that alcohol is a coping mechanism, but for me it has not been to a dangerous or detrimental level. That said, my hangovers are most uncomfortable with long-lasting deterioration in ability and that is something I need to consider when socialising in the evening.

While I have used this experience to demonstrate how alcohol can be an issue when working as a doctor, I feel I already have the personal abilities required to 'keep it in check'. I intend to enjoy all the benefits that qualifying offers without pickling my liver or harming a patient.

Finally, I am strongly against drink + driving and I intend to expand this belief to a complete drink + doctoring ban.

And then it hit me!

In my two weeks of shadowing, I can't say that there was one definite event that stood out. Our ward was closed for infection control reasons after an outbreak of diarrhoea and vomiting. Most of the patients of the ward had been discharged save a few who were essentially well but not well enough to actually go home. As I sat at the nurses' station copying out blood results into patient's notes and reading random bits in the *Oxford Handbook* I started to panic as it seemed there was no hope anything very exciting was going to happen – and what would I write about then? I have found that competitiveness is something that is quietly but very strongly encouraged throughout medical school and medicine in general. So what will I have to show for my shadowing week? Aaaarrgh!

The lack of activity made me think back to all the experiences I have had over the last five years, all the juicy ethical dilemmas, the amazing patients, the slightly strange patients, the family dynamics, the challenges that faced patients and doctors. And then it hit me – something major had already happened – medical school had happened to me or maybe through me and now it was nearly over. Taking stock of who I have become and what has contributed to how I am now, I came to realise how profoundly medical school had contributed to my personal development. Being exposed to patients and their families and so many other people every day is like being on an accelerated life learning curve. The days where you don't encounter something that challenges your vision of the world, your beliefs and emotions are few and far between. There is always a unique experience, a new way of looking at things, something else to learn, and something that no one had ever seen before. I have come into contact with so many people's lives and although I might not remember each and every one, I really believe that I have kept a part of them with me – they have all contributed, whether I was conscious of the fact or not, to who I am now.

The quiet contemplation had to stop for the moment, as it was time for a quick ward round with the registrar. During the round (I was effectively the PRHO for the ward as the real PRHO was affected by the dreaded D&V) something else became clear. I finally really felt I had a sense of purpose, that the work I was doing which many may regard as mundane was actually useful and necessary and I was REALLY contributing to the patients' care. Throughout medical school you usually feel that you are in someone's way, that you're just someone who clutters up ward rounds or clinics and takes up valuable time because you have to be taught. The student tends to put in a lot of hard work and try to be as useful as possible but he/she is limited by ability, understanding and the fact that people always say, 'You aren't here to help, you're here to learn'. I spent a lot of medical school feeling purposeless and unable to see the light at the end of the tunnel, constantly having to remind myself why I was doing this. But now, on the wards, I realised that I have almost arrived and all that one spends most of medical school working towards is now finally just a few steps away. Working on the wards as acting PRHO made me realise for the first time that I felt ready to start doing the job and it gave revision for finals meaning, as it would contribute to my competence as a doctor. Then my bleep went – 'Please come to the ward to see a patient who is deteriorating, her saturations are dropping,' said the nurse.

What ensued within me was a full-on 'fight or flight' response. After taking a deep breath I made my way to the ward with a heart rate of what felt like about

170 bpm and the words echoing in my head: 'Just remember the basics'. I went to see the patient and after another deep breath I did my basics – A–B–C–D – did some simple things like sit the patient up, gave her an oxygen mask with a rebreathing bag (her oxygen saturations actually came up!) and did some basic investigations; I wrote in the notes; discussed the patient with the registrar and asked the nurses to call me if she deteriorated again. As I left the ward, my heart rate still at least 120 bpm, I thought 'Oh my God! I can't believe I'm still alive or rather I can't believe the patient is still alive!' Once I had calmed down I became aware of several things.

1. Most patients you get called to see will probably not suddenly crash without warning (I think I've watched far too much *ER*) and even if they do you are not alone and you can call help quickly.
2. I have actually learned and am capable of thinking logically.
3. I can actually tap into knowledge I have acquired over the years and am able to apply that knowledge.
4. I know when I need help (I know when I'm out of my depth) and where to get it.

These things will undoubtedly seem incredibly obvious to anyone reading this. Medical school has taught me the important skills – what I've learned through shadowing is the fact that I didn't realise I actually had them until I had to apply them. As a medical student you are on the sidelines; you rarely are ACTUALLY in a position where you have to treat anyone. So although I know it will be just as nerve-racking the first time my real bleep goes off, I hope I'll be able to remember that I can think in a structured way and maybe my heart rate will only go up to 120 bpm rather than 170 bpm.

Overall, shadowing was a brilliant experience; not only do I have a much better idea about what I'll be doing but it also gave me a chance to actually start integrating the effect the last five years have had on me and how I have changed throughout them. They have influenced what I believe to be good and bad medical practice and shaped the doctor that I am becoming. In summary – I can't wait! Bring on finals!

'Only doing ward jobs': leaving professional puberty

At first, I thought a house officer shadowing course was a bit redundant. I thought I already knew what a house officer did. I thought I'd been shadowing them for years. In the second year they seemed to be the friendly face when consultants have been intimidating and distant figures. In the third and fourth year they were the people who used to be in the Galenicals sports teams, and in the fifth year they are our friends from halls who didn't intercalate. It seemed that I spent a lot of my time with house officers, and the time when I was *not* with them was when they were '*only doing ward jobs*'.

What I realised throughout the shadowing course was that although my social interaction was mostly with the juniors, I've actually spent most of my medical student 'career' shadowing consultants; shadowing them in clinic, theatre and on ward rounds, trying to assimilate some of their knowledge by passive osmosis. At this stage this is a bit silly, because I'm not going to be a consultant in four months time, but a house officer, and so house officer shadowing was entirely appropriate.

What I realised being surgically attached to a house officer during the course was that although the consultant provided instruction and direction it was the 'only doing ward jobs' which was really the leg work that made the firm move forward. Going round on ward rounds the consultant has always made decisions and I've always expected a magic wand to be waved and it to be done (maybe the consultant expects this as well). It is the house officer who does the ringing, the chasing, re-sites the venflon and enables the consultant to look like a magician.

It's hard work making things look easy; juggling patients' names, remembering jobs in the order they come on the wards, being efficient when everything in the system seems to work against you, running around all day until all the energy has drained out of your feet by the time you finish an hour later than you were supposed to.

But there is also a pride in it, a quiet satisfaction in the knowledge that if it weren't for you, it wouldn't happen. You are not supernumerary; a redundant extra person whose most useful contribution to the firm is opening and closing curtains on the ward round.

Being a medical student in the UK you struggle for a role. Friends who've studied History of Art, or other seemingly nebulous subjects, would envy us for our clearly defined role in the first year. But they graduated three years ago and now have rewarding (and well-paid) jobs in London. They have found their role in society but have left us behind in limbo, not 18-year-old teeny-boppers but not yet independent practitioners.

In other countries the medical training is also different. The courses are longer and students are apprentices. If there's an ECG that needs to be done, it's the medical student's job to do it, not a learning opportunity. This does however mean that their training is a lot longer. It only takes two goes to know how to do an ECG – in the French system you spend months and months doing it and book-work is postponed. But the European system does give you a role. In Holland the medical students went on strike because they felt that they weren't being taught and remunerated enough for the services they provided. If UK medical students went on strike I think the hospital would run more not less efficiently.

The loss of the apprenticeship system makes for more efficient and quicker training, but it does leave the students lacking an identity – a kind of second-wave professional adolescence – with all the insecurities that that entails.

What I've realised during the shadowing course is that 'only doing ward jobs' is what it's all about, or will be very soon. This shadowing course and our finals are our rite of passage into a new era with a new identity.

Tools of the job

Reality bites. My fortnight shadowing experience was to be in a general hospital, in surgery. The apprehension, however, remained. Would I like the job, the people, the place? Would they like me?

My guardian angel for the two weeks arrives in the impressive form of Ben with lots of reassurance that the job, while hard work, is rewarding and, with allowances for the inevitable paperwork, good fun too. And, lo and behold, a second guardian angel! This time the nurse specialist on the ward, Mary, who would be there with me in August. We clicked immediately. With such support, the fortnight couldn't be anything but a success.

First things first; the mess. Tea and coffee, check. Crunchy Nut Cornflakes, check. Comfy sofas and Sky TV, check. Then, of course, I had to be equipped with the tools of the job, namely Ben's bleep. Was that a look of relief as he handed it to me? A list of patients under our care was next, thankfully with only two outliers. I say thankfully as I was soon to discover the rabbit-warren, nonsensical nature of the layout of the hospital that seems designed to leave patients forgotten and newly qualified doctors pulling their hair out when lost in the maze.

Ward rounds were a hive of activity, especially Thursday when all three consultants were present. Writing in the notes during every ward round for two weeks has brought me to a decision. I need to marry someone who has a much shorter surname than mine! It is just too long to hurriedly sign off at the end of every entry, especially given the importance of legibility. Inevitably, the ward rounds generated lots of jobs, and, in the case of one particular consultant, numerous CT scans that needed to be done yesterday. Mary was therefore quick to fill me in on the names of radiologists that weren't averse to a bit of feminine charm. Urgent CT scan? No problem.

As medical students we are generally fortunate enough to have little contact with the piles of admin that are the remit of any house job. I was soon introduced, however, to the boxes of notes requiring discharge summaries to be completed. TTOs to be written, test results to be chased up or signed off. In actual fact, the novelty still had not worn off by the end of the fortnight but I was firmly assured that after a month on the job, the novelty would have worn thin to the point of non-existence. I am hoping that my many summers of temping as a medical secretary will hold me in good stead for efficient and accurate completion of such tasks. I have a very strong belief that the numerous members of 'behind-the-scenes' staff are pivotal in the smooth running of a hospital and I certainly do not plan to do anything that will get the consultants' secretaries off-side!

It was very satisfying to be introduced as the person who would be doing Ben's job in August. Five years of constantly being labelled as 'yet another medical student' has become rather tiresome. The shadowing experience engendered a special feeling of responsibility for the patients on the ward. Rather than the fleeting visits to find 'signs' or specific long cases in preparation for exams as might be considered the bread and butter of students with finals looming on the horizon, it highlighted the crucial role that a house officer can play in the front line of care for their patients. There is much more communication with relatives and liaison with other departments than is initially evident as a student, which is so pleasing to experience. Students are bombarded with 'medical humour' that may seem to predispose to a cavalier attitude to patients. I am so delighted that I will have room for a more holistic approach to patient care (even on a surgical ward!).

On a more technical note, it was the first time that I had actually been involved in management decisions. I have previously been quizzed on what to do in certain circumstances but never has my opinion been asked for, let alone valued. Maybe fluid balance decisions are deemed trivial in the general scheme of things (which I obviously realise they shouldn't be), but it truly meant something to be trusted to make the choice of whether a patient had a saline drip put up or not. Is that sad?

Pay Day Thursday. It was almost as if this fortnight had been planned to end on such a good evening. Can't wait until August.

The job IS comprehensible!

So it's early. And I'm awake. Definitely nervous. I don't know why it feels so much more daunting to walk onto the ward where (I hope) I will be working in a few months time. Perhaps it is the feeling that this fortnight is as close as I can get to having a sense of whether I can actually do the job that the last six years have been all about. What I really want is to be calm, sensible, confident, useful, helpful, and not end up writing up the wrong drug at the wrong dose for the wrong patient, missing the fourth attempt at a venflon on a needle-phobic patient, or completely forgetting about the three outliers that must be seen at the end of the consultant ward round. The list goes on.

So my house officer comes to meet me and we head off to what is his second ward round of what will be a busy day. It is fairly typical for surgery – a couple of minutes behind each set of curtains to hear about observations, temperatures, urine output, pain. But the third patient is only 46 and has just been told that he has disseminated intra-abdominal adenocarcinoma. His two children aged 10 and 12 do not know yet. Suddenly my fears and expectations of this morning seem to evaporate into the palest insignificance.

He has become one of those patients I will never forget. I will see my house officer providing regular contact, support and acting to ensure that other members of the team are involved. Sometimes we joked and smiled, sometimes we cried. It was an absolute confirmation that communication and the ability to listen *is* the vital skill in a good doctor. For the first time, it seemed to be obvious that it is only the house officer who can act as that point of contact in a surgical firm which, inevitably, spends most of its time in theatre and operates whirlwind ward rounds which rarely venture beyond hard, objective indicators of progress.

It made me think how easy it might be to get sucked into a system which is too stretched to look beyond our blinkered medicalised model of presenting complaint, and its narrow context of related symptoms, to the whole host of factors that make up a patient's important reality. I have always wanted to be the sort of doctor who will talk, listen, catch a glimpse of my patient's real life in the strange and impersonal hospital environment. And I would certainly hope that I will never be the kind who thinks that booking the CT scan in the next 10 minutes will make a patient feel much better than addressing their fears or explaining what is happening, either with patients or their relatives.

I also realised that my initial fear is really important. So many patients, and their relatives, end up in hospital and have their worlds blown apart by unexpected bad news, and the anonymity and lack of privacy in these fairly grim establishments can only worsen that feeling of fear of what the future may hold. Perhaps not forgetting how scary 'Day One' will inevitably be is a way of maintaining some kind of contact with at least part of our patients' hospital experience.

Shadowing has also been a great insight into how to learn on the job. It is not a process of passive absorption but requires you to recognise that you are not familiar with a particular aspect of the disease process or its management while it is being discussed and to ensure that you actively ask questions to find out more. The answers to those questions don't necessarily come from others in the medical profession but from colleagues across the multidisciplinary team. And it is also invaluable to see others practising – to learn both practical and communication skills that aid the detection and correct interpretation of the subtlest but most important of nuances. It was a real privilege to shadow an outstanding house officer.

As for that initial fear – it certainly hasn't gone and Day One will still represent a big step across the unspoken divide that protects students from any formal responsibility. But it is no longer a massive leap into the unknown – organising patient lists and ward rounds, booking investigations and gaining better understanding of how to access the breadth of skills and services which the multidisciplinary team offers suddenly makes the job comprehensible. Even the little things, like advance warning of which radiologists are better avoided when the Boss wants a CT done by yesterday and where the mess is, will make the early days much easier. Perhaps the most sensible way of putting the fear into perspective is by acknowledging that this is about doing your very best and learning at every opportunity to continuously improve.

Most of all, I have gained confidence in my own abilities, acknowledged that the first few weeks will be a real challenge and established the standards that I want to meet for the patients I am involved in the care of as a house officer next year. And I can't wait to see, do and learn more.

Doctors come and go; it's nurses who make the place

As you walk down the hill from the accommodation, the hulk of the building that is the hospital looms above you. On my first morning I stopped, looked up, and took in what, exams pending, could be my home for the next year. Events that take place within its four walls, within the city around it, are going to shape the biggest transition of my life.

Of course you felt the same when you started university, but you had a huge group of people in the same boat. There is no routine (apart from lectures), you and your new comrades, out experiencing life away from the family nest, build your own lifestyle, your own daily pattern.

From the beginning of August, I will be starting out with a new group of friends, ready and willing (well, nearly) to experience the next stage. This time, however, we will be superimposed on to a system that has been working effectively for years, resilient to six-monthly tides of people like us, slipping into the routine. In any other profession or company it wouldn't work. Such a workforce turnover would be counter-productive. However, we have trained for five years, getting closer to the starting gate, waiting for it to be released and to fill in the gaps left by those six months ahead of you. While being a shadow I realised why this can happen – nurses. They carry on regardless, providing a seamless service to patients, as the newest group of doctors begin to establish themselves in the background.

The ward I was to shadow on holds a full capacity of 40 patients, a mixture of old and new, and those trapped inside due to Norwalk virus. The first day was spent meeting and greeting those belonging to my consultant. My house officer carrying out his round introduced me as the lady soon to be doing his job. At first I ignored the words as I was expecting them. I knew what he was saying and why – this was the recommended description for us shadows – but then I actually thought about them. It really wasn't long until I actually was going to be the doctor, checking on the welfare of patients, helping, organising and communicating, inside and outside the hospital.

As the first week progressed, the awe did not even begin to fade. As a student I had never spent so long on one ward. You would go and see your friends, see who they recommended you 'look at', go to clinic, have a long coffee, etc. Now I began to see how well the ward really works, and how much a house officer is involved in the big team, the clerks, nurses, physiotherapists, occupational therapists and dieticians. You no longer just know the patients you've clerked. You build a rapport with everyone, you are comfortable with approaching most, smiling acknowledgement, making chit chat, informing them of progress and things planned, patients and staff alike. They respond differently; you are different. You no longer have the expression of a hunter, checking people only for their use in helping you to learn and pass your exams. It is refreshing, it is rewarding, you have become an influential part of their hospital experience and they have become so much a part of yours. Every day there are new faces, but everything keeps flowing.

I began to know some patients very well; the highs and lows of not just their illness but of their lives became my knowledge. I began to contribute to the team, adding pieces to the jigsaw that is every patient's story. One gentleman had a post-lunch 'dip' in his lucidness and developed a tremor. This was only witnessed by myself and his wife, so I became the main witness, describing it for the rest of the team, helping everyone to add bits to the pictures they were all painting of the patient. It felt good to be a useful part of the round, my opinion elicited and trusted. It gave me the incentive to work hard and get on to the next rung of the ladder, have a group that were 'my patients', not in a selfish way, but in a protective, proud way. I would be included within my firm.

My most memorable incident reminded me that, however confident we feel, we are all fallible. One ward round, blood gases were needed urgently on a patient. I was excused to obtain the sample and bring back the results. I went off, a spring in my step that my technical skills were trusted. I set up the kit, went and introduced myself to the patient and his wife, explained my position and why I needed this sample. He consented, giving me his wrist. I smiled thankfully, and again at his wife as she kindly offered any assistance – that was until she finished her offer with 'I used to be a nurse'. Suddenly I felt insecure, the confidence draining, as if she could see through the cool, professional exterior I hoped to be projecting. They both knew I was a final year student, but she actually knew what it meant. She had seen hundreds before me, young students and fresh-faced doctors, having a go at being useful.

I turned to the task, worrying that the longer I took, any fumbling that took place, would increase the rising ebb of fear that I assumed was bubbling inside them. I looked at the medial aspect of his wrist, feeling the gentle pulse beneath. I prayed to strike oil as I pushed the needle deep. I looked down, relief flooding my senses as red liquid surged into the syringe. I leant across for the cotton wool, my fingers coming back empty. The premature relief was replaced by a rising 'oh bugger'. I scanned around, feeling as if the level rising in the syringe was like a pressure reading on a thermostat, about to blow. Suddenly a box of tissues shone out across the table; quickly using one to cover the puncture site, I applied pressure. What had happened was minor, but I explained I had forgotten gauze. As I went to get some, I reflected on the rollercoaster of emotion I had just been through. I had put pressure on myself by thinking too much about what his wife was thinking – a mountain out of a molehill situation – and soon realised that a year of this would turn me grey! I questioned my house officer on how you get over this, being reassured that you soon relax as you become more practised and natural.

Chatting with the patient and his wife later made me understand that we may feel naïve and inexperienced, trying so hard to fit in, but that isn't a bad thing. Very few staff look down upon this. They have seen it in hundreds before, and realise we aren't born fully trained. Learning by experience, some of these mistakes (luckily mainly minor) are all part of our transition. It makes us better, and she told me how they all became quite proud of their house doctors, as they watch them mature over their six months. She reminded me that we are all different but actually all the same; we just can't look past our own job experiences. It can be a turbulent ride but they know this and will support us in their own discrete ways. It usually isn't as bad as we are feeling, and all our friends are going through exactly the same thing.

By the end of the two weeks, I had learned so much, silly things like to look at what ward you are entering (as they all look pretty similar when you are on them), to wear comfortable shoes for all the stair climbing (perhaps a few gym sessions needed before August as well!), to carry forms around with you to save time, and of course how the consultant likes his coffee!

We sat on the last day, the whole team enjoying doughnuts. I looked around, sad to be going, glad to be coming back. The nurses wished me well; the 'looking forward to seeing you in August' may have just been polite, but it made me leave with a smile, the prospect of coming back a good one. I felt supported, knowing I was going to be helped out throughout my year, to be brought along and matured, to have friends, on and off the ward, involved in my highs and lows.

Three people with HIV

My shadowing week has been hugely encouraging for me; both in terms of clinically 'learning the ropes' (and in some cases finding out where the ropes were in the first place), and for my own personal development. It was another stuttering step from the cocoon of studentship to the fragile butterfly of the pre-registration year. Thankfully, I found myself able to reflect on many incidents during my stay. Three memories stand out, united by the differing challenges of people with HIV.

HIV – my fears

On my first day shadowing my future job, I met more HIV-positive people than I had ever chatted to in a clinical context before. Some were heartbreakingly ill, two were dealing with the burden of a recent positive diagnosis and one man was so clouded by dementia that the diagnosis had to be rebroken to him daily. The first time I took blood from a (known) HIV-positive patient is a vivid memory.

I felt comfortable with him, and my hand–eye skills – but nothing makes you reassess your technique more than the irrational sweating of 'what if'? What if I sneeze and needle-stick myself? Will I go from supporting this frail human being, to hating him for what would essentially be my mistake? I felt reassured by being able to share these dark childish fears with my house officer, who offered me both practical risk-reduction advice and anxiety reassurance. She was right; your levels of care for a higher-risk procedure remain at a maximum, despite your apprehension ebbing away with practice. By the end of my week I found myself hugging an HIV-positive lady from Malawi, and I realised that I had been able to re-inject the human back into 'these patients'.

HIV – sympathy

My second reflection is on my feelings surrounding a seriously ill gentleman. I walked into the side-room on the ward round, to meet a thin-faced chap who was gasping for breath. He had four chest drains in, and was so emaciated as to make a stick man jealous. My bubbly heart sank, as I recognised the sober tone in the team. The man struggled to pull his head in my direction and nodded a dignified 'hello'. I stood there feeling inadequate, my doubts of 'what am I doing here?' now being tempered with 'what would I be doing here next year?' He was only 31, closer in age to my house officer and me than to anyone else in our extensive team – yet he looked frailer than I remember Grampy, and almost as old. My heart really melted for this poor patient; he must have been seriously ill for too long a time before reaching hospital. On questioning, he admitted that he had no close friends, besides his Mum. My consultant went back to the bedside. Here he broke the news to this skeletal but fighting man that he was HIV positive. I was genuinely impressed by his empathy, compassion and straight talking.

Our consultant asked the gasping man his knowledge of HIV and AIDS, and built his message on that base of facts and beliefs. It seemed that our patient had no easily recognised risk factors; however, as we were leaving, our battling man called back, 'Doctor, doctor'. There was then just the wheeze of high flow oxygen as we turned towards him, and he regained his mettle for each stolen word. 'I was raped, by a man, when I was sixteen,' he deliberately spat out – despite the hindrance of the mask. The mechanism of how this guy had developed his illness would make no difference to his treatment, but in that moment, as a person, I couldn't help but melt with sympathy for him. Over a coffee, I was pleased that the doctor I was shadowing had also felt the same. It was comforting to discover that 'real medicine' doesn't automatically harden the heart.

HIV – communication skills

My third account is a reflection of learning from the actions of my house officer and her team. On our ward was a lady with HIV admitted for palliative care, but her dependence on methadone left her very drowsy. Her only solace was chain-smoking, but her lack of mobility made nursing her solely on the patio impractical. It was pragmatically decided to prevent her from smoking by removing her cigarette lighter and occasionally allow supervised smoking.

Unfortunately, during my placement with the team, a terrifying and regrettable incident occurred. A nurse not used to the ward allegedly left the room while supervising the cigarette – only to be called back in by the screams of the patient who was in flames. It transpires that the oxygen prongs were left flowing (but beside her pillow), fuelling this horrific scene. The lady's burns were more superficial than you would expect, but over an extensive area on her left side.

I was impressed at how all the staff were able to disguise their guilt/blaming of her to treat her burns with the care and sympathy they deserved. I watched my house officer add to her list of jobs for Monday morning, communicating with all the appropriate people. Additionally, she had to assist the ward manager, liaise with medical photography and then deal understandingly with the 17 members of the patient's family who visited the ward (as they had originally planned to take her out as a 'last wish'). Uppermost were her duties to the patient's health, yet she also had an obligation to represent the manager and the trust, while still being the patient's and relative's advocate. I didn't envy the position she found herself in, but admired the confident open way she was able to listen and offer support. I was also reassured by the amount of constructive assistance she received from the senior members of the team.

Conclusion

To conclude, I have presented my reflections on three people with HIV and the emphatically different challenges they presented to me and my house officer in my shadowing week. Learning is best gained from experience, and I was privileged to be in a position where there were abundant poignant situations to convince me that my first three months in my new job will be the antithesis of boring. I honestly feel more prepared, if anything can prepare you, for the challenge of being a pre-registration house officer.

Breaking bad news badly

It was while walking down a silent corridor at 3 o'clock in the morning to an unknown patient on an unknown ward that the true implications of what qualifying will hold for us hit me. At the same time I felt relief that not everything that we will face will actually be new to us. While the line 'I'm just a student' will no longer hold true and we will have to re-site that venflon or write up some fluids, I feel prepared for my PRHO year and found the shadowing week hugely beneficial.

The course involves close observation of the present PRHO while always thinking about what you would do if you were in their shoes. The incident that I have chosen to write about remains at the forefront of my mind, because I think that it highlights the transition from student to doctor, from learning the ideal to the reality.

My incident involved one of the medical outlying patients who came in on the consultant's take. My PRHO had therefore not met the patient before. It was getting towards the end of the post-take ward round and the enthusiasm of the team was depleted. We reached the last bed of the bay and saw a gentleman asleep, looking extremely jaundiced. The man awoke as the whole team crowded around the bed and the PRHO struggled to relay the history from the illegible notes. The consultant latched onto the CT result which indicated that a mass was seen in the head of the pancreas. The consultant then told the patient that he had cancer. Just like that; no warnings, despite there being no tissue diagnosis and in front of a group of strangers. He then briefly stated that a stent could be placed to relieve some of the symptoms and walked onto the next patient. The PRHO who had been scribbling in the notes looked up and found herself left in the cubicle with the patient crying in front of her. We both felt completely torn, appalled at the situation and yet faced with an unknown distraught patient and a consultant who wanted to finish the round.

I actually felt that the PRHO dealt with the situation very well and professionally. She offered a few minutes of sympathy and reassurance to the patient, promising to come back and explain the diagnosis properly when the ward round had finished. She then managed to catch one of the nurses and explain the situation to them so hopefully the patient wasn't alone for too long.

I chose this example as I feel it raises several important points for discussion. First, I experienced the effects of breaking bad news badly. I don't know the consultant's reasons for being so abrupt and insensitive – surely time and pressures are not so extreme so as to deny a dying man five minutes of explanations and reassurance. This was real-life medicine and the most important skill we have got to develop. We must adapt a strategy for ensuring that we put what we have learned into our practice, however stressed or busy. Real medicine is full of 'in theory, in an ideal world'. While being realistic and getting the job done, we should try and build on all the training we have had in communication skills to ensure that this scenario doesn't happen again.

On reflection, maybe the consultant didn't realise that he had let the patient down. I remember feeling outraged at the time with his attitude but I was not going to question my future consultant. Perhaps I should have?

This case also highlights a problem I noticed over the shadowing – the lack of continuity. The house officers no longer do takes for their consultants and the patients are scattered all over the hospital. This fact exacerbated the situation as the house officer could not even predict the patient's response to the bad news. This stresses the importance of handover, legible note writing and involving the nursing staff before talking to the patients.

The importance of teamwork is once again stressed as the PRHO recognised that the nurses have a key role in offering support to the patients. During our first year, we will probably not have to break much bad news ourselves but we will be a vital part of the team in helping patients and relatives to come to terms with their grief.

While I would have preferred this incident not to have occurred, it was a useful learning point for me as I was able to observe how the PRHO handled the situation and the painful effects of badly explained news which will encourage me to always try to get it right.

In conclusion, I thoroughly enjoyed the shadowing experience and it has given me more confidence for starting the job in August. I learned all the odd jobs that you never see as a student such as administering the first dose of a drug and certifying somebody as dead. I hope I will not now be phased by the routine jobs I will be asked to do. It was also encouraging to see for myself the support you get as a junior. All the ward rounds are conducted with the SHO and the patients you clerk on take have to be reviewed. The final message that clearly came across was: 'If in doubt, ASK!'

A medical practitioner in my own right

Shadowing the PRHO in the NHS trust that I will be working for in August was an altogether valuable experience for many reasons. I learned many practical things such as where all the request forms are kept, where the mess is and how to use the telephones (altogether modern, not like any other hospital I have been on attachment in!). I learned how to get to the x-ray department and to theatres without losing my way and I mastered how to get into the computer system to check blood results without barring the person whose password I was using. I made myself known to the important people on my future ward – the sisters, the nurse practitioners, the ward clerks and, oh yes, the consultants too.

Everyone seemed very friendly and I am truly looking forward to getting stuck in. The overriding thoughts in my mind during the whole week were: 'I'm going to be one of them in a few months! This is going to be me!' Kathy Feest's words echoed, 'Do what they do'. One night my PRHO informed me that I must not be late the following morning as all the consultants would be doing a huge joint ward round with the entire firm. This was the first time that I would be meeting them, so I was quite nervous.

On the ward in the morning, I made the effort to be extra smiley and helpful. As I shook each of the three consultants' hands, I was thinking 'These are my bosses, I must please them, I must use them as mentors and role models'. As we steered the entourage around the beds, the nurses became twitchy because we couldn't close the curtains around each bed due to the large number of people on the ward round. Like my PRHO, I rolled my eyes heavenward too, belittling their concern.

It was OK when the surgeon was just enquiring after their wound and pain relief. When he lifted up pyjama tops to examine abdomens, I started to feel a bit twitchy myself and looked away as much as possible, even though efforts were made to maintain the patients' dignity with strategically placed blankets. The bit that really got to me was going to see a rather frail elderly lady who had just had an endoscopy for dysphagia. An oesophageal cancer was discovered and an attempt to place an oesophageal stent had been made at the initial endoscopy but was unsuccessful.

Instead of ordering away the unnecessary onlookers from the bed and breaking the news of her cancer slowly, quietly and gently, the surgeon proceeded to tell her that 'We have found a malignant growth in your oesophagus and we tried to deploy a stent to relieve your dysphagia but it failed to deploy properly so we are going to try again but with a longer Flamingo this time. Any questions? No? OK, good, see you tomorrow.' And bear in mind that this was with the curtains open, 10 people observing and no relatives with the patient. I was horrified at this and felt desperately sorry for the elderly lady. No doubt all she would have understood of the surgeon's statement was that she had cancer and that the doctors' efforts to relieve her symptoms had failed. How frightening for her!

As a medical student, I am very aware of patients' dignity and a right to privacy. I even pull the curtains around the bed when I approach someone to take blood or put in a cannula! However, on going away and thinking about this incident, I became upset with myself for not suggesting that the curtains be pulled around the bed or that some of us leave, once I realised what was going on. This would not be new for me, as I have done it on countless other ward rounds and have been praised afterwards for thinking of the patient's feelings first. Being a medical student, you learn to take on the routine and, to some extent, the practices of the firm to which you are attached. You also learn to respect the patient's dignity as part of examination technique and how to break bad news in a sympathetic manner. The thing was that I became too preoccupied with being 'just like them'.

I have realised that becoming a PRHO is not about imitating my superiors and 'doing what they do'; it is about becoming a medical practitioner in my own right, with my own routine, my own practices where only I am responsible for these. I just hope that, in the future, a temporarily overwhelmed medical student does not witness me doing anything quite so insensitive.

Giving people good news is easy, isn't it?

In the middle of a busy business ward round many of the tasks may seem at best uninspiring and, at worst, somewhat mundane. One Thursday, having seen several patients undergoing relatively straightforward convalescence from routine elective operations, we visited the rather anxious lady in the last bay on the ward.

Several days earlier she had undergone an anterior resection of the bowel to remove a tumour. The histology result on the resected tissue took rather longer than expected to return from the laboratory. That morning it had finally appeared on the computer.

The report read: '*Non-invasive tubulo-villous adenoma. Serosal edge inflamed but not involved in tumour. Excision margins show no evidence of tumour. Several lymph nodes sent in sample – none infiltrated.*'

The first reactions of the SHO and house officer (actually a year four SHO doing a locum) were, respectively, 'Oh, right, Duke's A' and 'Well, it looks like we got it then'. With that, they turned and carried on with their preparations for the ward round.

Having had recent experience of a family friend in a similar situation, my thoughts were 'We must go and tell her, she'll be so pleased', envisioning a contented grin spreading across her face. My second thought was 'Thank heavens we don't have to tell her it's bad/has spread/needs re-operating' and mentally switched off the 'breaking bad news' train of thought that had been forming in my mind.

Well – giving people good news is easy, isn't it?

So, there we are: registrar, SHO, 'house officer', myself, and a staff nurse gathered round the end of the bed. I must admit that, up until now, I had been a little distracted; quietly excited at the news we had for this lady, who had asked about her 'sample' every time I'd seen her for the previous four days. We ran through the usual routine of temperature, blood pressure, pulse, wound status, appetite and bowel function. All the time she was looking increasingly restless. I was desperate to tell her what I knew, and every second that she wasn't told was beginning to feel like an eternity to me. Quite what she must have been feeling, I can't imagine.

Then, utterly without context or even looking up from the notes, the registrar announced, 'We meant to tell you, that bit of bowel we took out …' The patient looks expectant. An ominous pause follows (presumably while the registrar translates the report into English) and the patient's face gradually falls. The 'house officer' is, by now, looking slightly smug. He knows what's coming and he's sure she's going to like it.

'Well, it's like this,' the registrar continued, 'the problem was confined to the piece of bowel that we took out, and wasn't in the lymph nodes.' And that, he thought, was that. I was just thinking how I could, or would, have done it differently, when there came a loud sob.

Bemused looks darted between the surgeons. This lady, perfectly intelligent, sound of mind and hearing, had just been told that her malignant tumour had been completely removed. Although none of us would dare use the word cure, that was in effect what had been said. So why was she upset?

Of course, she wasn't. They were tears of joy and relief. But her reaction took us all by surprise. When I see a patient cry, the instant reaction is that something terrible must have happened to them. Either they are in pain, or the medical profession, by going about its normal work, has completely shattered their life. In other words, something has gone desperately wrong. Not so this time. Despite the tears from the patient, I felt my spirits lift. This was what I had chosen to do medicine for. To make that positive influence in someone's life, and to experience more fully the scope of the human state.

However, it also got me thinking about aspects of medical education. We sit in numerous workshops on the breaking of bad news but we don't get sessions on conveying positive messages; they are considered easy. However, they may not be so straightforward. This patient, in my opinion, didn't have her diagnosis well explained, and the tears could easily have been because she had misunderstood the message. Thankfully they weren't. Also, none of us had taken into account the fact that she was so pre-occupied with the expectation of being told that her disease had spread that she could easily have heard the wrong message.

The setting may also have been inappropriate. We are all aware of the need for privacy when breaking bad news but what about good news? The rest of the bay saw this poor woman burst into tears, and they all instantly assumed that they knew what had been said. It is worth bearing in mind quite how much the rest of the bay listen to consultations and know about each other's conditions.

The same techniques should be borne in mind when any important news is delivered to patients – it is not only in the breaking of bad news that communication skills are tested and where the opportunity exists to seriously disturb patients.

It is as important to learn to deliver good news competently and sensitively, as it is bad. In both cases, there are no second chances; they are both life-changing events.

Words and silences: I'm sorry

Language is both the vehicle and the obstacle. One so wishes that one could use a medium that is more invisible than language. We have freighted words with too many meanings, so one word does not mean the same thing to everybody. Words that are intended to unite end up dividing, and those that are intended to be innocent actually end up being insulting. The difficulty here is how to use words in a way that transcends words: to get to what words are, at the end of the day, trying to get to, which is silence, stillness and that resonating chamber. The final destination of 'words' is to render themselves invisible, to be removed into a higher state which is thought, and therefore the condition of being. It is a strange paradox. Everywhere I turn, I hear people talking about language as if it were brick, as if it were a thing that is never absorbed into the spirit. It is not a physical thing, it is abstract marks on a page, it is a set of sounds. It is intangible. The only effect it has on us is that it resonates in us. That's it, and after you've read, the repercussions change and continue. It's one of the most extraordinarily dynamic processes, much more complex than the ripples when you throw stones into water.

I think we need more of the wordless in our lives. We need more stillness, more of a sense of wonder, a feeling for the mystery of life.

We began before words, and we will end beyond them.

I've thought a lot about words over the last two weeks. I didn't intend to. I intended to learn who to pester in the radiology department to get investigations done. I intended to learn how to get an arterial blood gas and put venflons in with finesse as well as under duress, but mostly I intended to make myself appear not entirely riddled with ineptitude in front of my new surgical consultants, registrars and the nurses on the wards.

I sit here at the end of two weeks and, without a doubt, the most valuable thing I have achieved is that I have learned to say, 'I'm sorry'.

During my PRHO shadowing, I was following a wonderful PRHO. He was incredibly organised, very dedicated and highly intelligent. The guy walked around, overflowing with so much medical knowledge that it practically leaked out of him. He would turn his head to look at you and unintentionally five medical facts would come flying out. One of those unique types who would ask me in all seriousness things like: 'So tell me, where does the word "warfarin" come from? Did you know that the way warfarin was discovered is fascinating – have a guess how they found out about it? I'll give you a clue, it has something to do with clover!' When he wasn't exuding medical facts, he was encouraging me to put in venflons and check blood results, which was just what I needed to get to grips with the job.

'Great guy,' I thought at the end of my first few days. Other PRHOs agreed. Apparently people were in awe of him. Even the other final year students who were shadowing their medical PRHOs would come up to me and say, 'Do you know this surgical PRHO who is meant to be amazing; apparently he knows everything, the medical SHOs were talking about him at lunchtime?' He worked hard and did his job to the best of his ability. The rest spoke for itself.

But what he could do that really made an impression on me was that he knew how to say 'I'm sorry' and he said it well. It's something we say a lot as medical students. 'I'm sorry for slowing down your clinic.' 'I'm sorry for not knowing the 137 causes of unilateral ptosis.' 'I'm so sorry for the massive haematoma I've just caused you while trying to take your blood.' I've become pathologically apologetic over the last five years. It's not until now that I've learned how to say it and what it really means.

My PRHO knew, and I don't even think he knows that he knows. But he does. The realisation came to me when we went to see a patient with a bed sore, who had been given an air pressure mattress. She wasn't happy with this and was crying out to anyone who would listen to ask the doctors to change it back. We went to see her to explain. He listened to her for what seemed like a long while. My first red flag that something was unusual was that he was absolutely silent while listening to her. No pacifying 'hmmms', no dismissive 'yes, I knows'. All he did was listen to her while looking directly at her, and then say, with the most gentle caring tone I've ever heard, 'I'm sorry'. He paused for a bit to let her absorb that apology, and then continued to explain why she had to have the mattress. Watching him felt like one of those surreal moments in time, perhaps akin to that moment people talk about before blacking out or having a fit … things go quiet, things slow down … your vision becomes tunnelled and absolutely focused … and then you come to. He did it again while I was shadowing him and, again, it felt odd to watch. (I know now that 'odd' feeling was the feeling of being really moved.)

We went to take an arterial blood gas sample from a lady. My PRHO had difficulty with it. He tried once without success, so he tried again. She was being very brave, and holding her pain in to herself, but then she just couldn't take it any more and just started to cry. He stopped his attempt immediately. He took his gloves off and let her recover, all the while looking straight at her with a pained look on his face. Again, he said, 'I'm really sorry.' I think he must have said it a couple of times, very gently but directly and full of sincerity.

I realised at that moment that on the whole, when I apologise to patients, to consultants, to other people, I'm apologising for myself, for my lack of skills or knowledge, for my error in judgement. My PRHO made me see that my focus is completely misguided. When I apologise, the focus is about me. When he apologises, the focus is on the other person who is suffering. That is the way it should be.

We are all taught to be careful with words. We've been to the communication skills sessions. We've bought the communications skills t-shirts. It is the implications of the words we use which are often lost to us. Perhaps that is what the writer means when he talks about needing to use words to transcend words. It is about what you say inbetween silences and how that connects us as human beings. As doctors we deal with ordinary people dealing with sometimes extraordinary pressures. We use words to clarify and to explain. 'Communicate with your patients and colleagues,' we're told. I think I'll follow my PRHO's philosophy of using less words, better. Words are there to heal as well. I know that now.

At times we forget how difficult it must be

> When you tell your trouble to your neighbour you present him with a part of your heart. If he possesses a great soul, he thanks you; if he possesses a small one, he belittles you. (Kahlil Gibran)

There are so many things that I have learned from my shadowing experience of a surgical pre-registration house officer post. Some have been practical, such as knowing how to write a prescription chart and request tests out of hours, which will smooth out the transition from an admittedly rather nervous, uncertain student to assertive and competent doctor. However, I feel that at the end of the shadowing I walk away with a lot more than this. There is one particular lesson that I consider precious and will try to carry with me for the rest of my professional life. This is what makes the PRHO that I shadowed not a good doctor but a great one.

She believes in listening to a patient; not just their medical history but also their concerns and thoughts with regard to their treatment. She understands how difficult such revelations sometimes are and how privileged we are as doctors to be told things that patients are at times hesitant to reveal even to their loved ones, and she acknowledges this to the patient. After the morning ward round and urgent jobs were completed, my PRHO and I would do a quick ward round of patients that she was concerned about. These include patients who are anxious, depressed and confused as to their current situation. Also her own personal concerns about a patient would be enough to prompt her to have a chat with them. She believes this gives patients a chance to voice their feelings away from a sometimes intimidating and time-pressed ward round. There were many examples of *good listening* over the eight days. The following is one of them.

One of our patients was a diabetic wheelchair user with advanced retinopathy who had had an above-knee amputation some years ago due to peripheral vascular disease. This time he was in hospital due to infected ulcers that were failing to heal on his remaining leg. Initially it was decided that his management be conservative with rest, elevation and daily bathing. Unfortunately his ulcers showed no signs of resolution and due to an element of large vessel disease he was offered the option of balloon angioplasty during the morning's ward round. He immediately started crying, refusing to have the operation. The consultant tried to impress on him the fact that this was not a decision that had to be made straight away and that he should voice what his concerns were, but the patient refused to elaborate and turned his back to the team.

My house officer and I returned later, introduced ourselves and perched on his bed. The PRHO started by simply asking him how he was feeling that day and then stayed quiet. He slowly started opening up, building up momentum as he spoke about his fears of whether he would ever return to the independence he had enjoyed prior to being admitted and his fear of what would happen to him. She stayed quiet and attentive throughout, gently holding his hand when he started crying as tacit acknowledgement of his pain, but not once succumbing to the temptation to interject with a comment.

When he finally fell silent, I realised that this might have been if not the only time, then one of very few times he had had a chance to express himself during his stay. She then said something that surprised me: 'Thank you, at times we forget how difficult it must be.' I think it was the sincere way in which she said this that made him answer honestly when she then asked directly what his fears were about the angioplasty. He revealed that he recalled the prolonged, excruciating and burning pain he had endured when he had had the procedure done to his other leg. At the time he felt he was given no control and was not being listened to by the radiologist. The procedure had been unsuccessful and he ended up with an above-knee amputation. He was petrified of going through the same pain and was far happier with having his leg cut off. We relayed this back to the SHO and registrar and he was booked in for a below-knee amputation.

Although we will not be making big decisions in a patient's management, our role in guiding what those decisions are, through listening, is significant. What my PRHO showed me was that our strength as junior doctors is that we are seen as more approachable while having enough knowledge to address many patient anxieties and enquiries. Therefore, as I get ready for my first day as a PRHO and go through my tick list of things to remember; stethoscope, bleep, badge, tourniquet, pen and pen torch, *Oxford Handbook of Clinical Medicine*, loose change and survival kit for ward round, I'll be sure to also remember to listen. After all what is the point of trying to *effectively* manage someone if you do not know exactly what the full biological, social and psychological aspects of their problems are?

How sure is sure enough?

Hospital ward – Monday 10 pm

Arterial blood gases (ABGs) are a useful measure of the severity of acute respiratory conditions. I have, in the course of clinical medical experience, attempted a probable figure of 150 ABGs, and been successful at the first attempt almost 100% of the time recently. I hope I am not conceited, and will remain so post-qualification, carefully checking my walk and talk for swagger.

It was quite a surprise, therefore, to find myself boasting about my ability to perform a successful ABG! My shadow-casting PRHO took it in the same quiet, happy, unsurprised way that he appears to take to everything on the ward. I quickly shut up, feeling a fool for having found myself boasting like a seven year old with 500 football stickers. The matter of my 'prodigal ABG gift' was forgotten, but not by me and not by the PRHO.

Bedside manners

The PRHO for medicine was on late on call, so I was the late on-call PRHO for medicine shadowing medical student. We arrived on the ward, where the PRHO was expecting a board full of jobs. Surprisingly there were only two, a chart to be rewritten and an ABG! The PRHO suggested that I do the ABG, and I tried not to swagger into the clinical stores. To my dismay I found that the hospital had a different ABG kit than I had been used to. In this hospital there were no ready-made packs, with pre-heparinised barrels and nice rubber bungs to poke the needle into. It's a hard life with no heparin, no resistance-less syringes, and big blue needles. *Why* had I boasted about my flagship investigation?

Through the assistance of the nursing staff I found myself with the correct cardboard tray and bits and pieces. I located the patient, a calm but breathless on oxygen, 65-year-old woman, surrounded by two female relatives, the younger of whom appeared to behave in a developmentally delayed way. This younger member of the family in particular found my arrival, complete with intent and cotton wool, fairly alarming. She wanted to stay and look after her grandmother. However, I tried to reassure everyone, telling them about what I wanted to do and why. The patient was evidently flavour of the month on levels eight and nine, battle decorated with cotton wool balls, like a fence post in a sheep field. Her hands were deformed by rheumatoid arthritis, and I had difficulty positioning her, as-yet unused, wrist comfortably.

Uneasily I managed to get what I confidently felt was arterial blood, despite having to draw on the syringe plunger, which had not been necessary before with resistance-less syringes. The patient commented that the sample looked very dark, and that she had some sort of blood disorder. I waited with her until all bleeding had stopped and returned to the clinical room to load a special '12-pound-a-go' blood gas cartridge.

Twelve pounds!

In the clinical room a nurse showed me how to fill the cartridge and get the machine to read it. The first attempt was not successful, and the oxygen was not read. I filled another cartridge with some more blood that was left. This time the machine did not read it at all, and a nurse reminded me that each single use cartridge cost 12 pounds. The PRHO asked me if I was *sure* it was arterial blood.

I wanted to say I was sure but:

- this was a difficult attempt
- getting very dark blood
- using unfamiliar equipment
- some of which wasn't working properly.

I wanted to say I was sure because of:

- the patient
- and most of all the PRHO
- not hurting the patient again
- not wanting to waste more time
- and wasting 24 pounds so far.

So I said I was pretty sure but didn't know about being sure enough, and explained my difficulty giving a yes/no answer.

Whether I was sure enough or not would not have made much of a difference in the end; it appeared to be a mechanical fault, and we ended up taking another sample anyway. However, being openly asked how confident I was about something I was claiming to have done made me reflect upon *what* makes me sure.

After some thought it appeared that the upper list of doubts, now and in the future, may be remedied by experience. The lower list of reasons to be sure should only ideally contain previous experience and anatomical knowledge. Thus experience past, present and future could be the answer to the question of: how sure is sure enough?

The job

The explanation is certainly an over-simplification. Only experience stood out as a motivating force not manipulated by time, place, emotional or physical state or ego. Through careful understanding of our own knowledge, knowledge only obtainable through personal clinical experience, can we be sure of ourselves as we practise clinical skills and decision making. 'The Three Ps of Perfect Performance' (as told to me by someone, once upon a time) include practice as well as preparation and patience. Incorporating these ideas daily will be a challenge, but could be useful guides in many situations. Hopefully the fourth P, for panic, will not scare me into being 'damn sure', or blind me to the subjective experience of being sure enough to be sure.

Silent words

Preface

> Stertis adhuc? laxumque caput conpage solute oscitat hesternum
> Dissutis undique malis? Est aliquid quo tendis, et in quod derigis arcum? (Persius, *Satire III*)
> [Are you still snoring? Is your slack head almost snapped on its stalk, with your face unzipped by the yawns earned in yesterday's debaucheries? Do you have any goals in life? Is there any point to your life?]

I found choosing one event difficult. In my experience, the shadowing week represented the qualifying heats to a race that I will begin after my graduation. It was both an opportunity to gauge the environment into which I would enter, but also to gauge myself in that environment.

Clinical medicine is not a new concept, but I have never been as ill prepared for an attachment as I was for the shadowing week. Of course there have been many opportunities to follow and assist pre-registration house officers, but never to the extent that I was privileged to experience while undertaking this part of the course.

During my time at the trust I felt that some of the key objectives that I hoped to have achieved would have been to grasp some of the fundamental aspects of practical survival as part of a clinical team. Although these are modest goals when compared to the overall learning experiences that have culminated in the last five years of intensive teaching and learning, they were, nonetheless, challenging.

I cannot deny the impact that this experience has had upon me. It was with great difficulty that I felt I could express these feelings – not least in such a limited volume. If I gained one thing from the shadowing placement, it was a greater understanding of myself; especially my limitations. The most significant of these related to a situation involving a lady with diagnosed pseudo-bulbar palsy, resulting in inability to either swallow or speak. I was deeply touched by this patient and her relatives. With the help of the team with which I was based, I was able to come to a better understanding of a holistic approach to the management of a patient who had been perfectly independent and active only six months ago, but who had since rapidly deteriorated.

These situations helped me develop interpersonal skills, as well as cement my personal opinions about *dignity* and *quality of life*; things that I had long considered abstract. Naturally, this experience invited the extensive clerical role of the PRHO; however, it was the daily patient and relative interaction that I felt I really began to understand in preparation for the honour of treating people in the future.

After much thought, I hoped to convey my experiences (including fears and elation) in as subjective a way as possible, not just from me, but subjective in interpretation, since, as with any personal experience, there will never be a perfect explanation or derivation, so I hope I have created an impression from which some understanding of *my* experience may be shared. For this opportunity, I thank you.

Silent Words

Too short my voyage seems to have brought me here …
My keys soon taken, I sought out my room.
The air mild, I am still spared from its heat:
Both hands, closed hard, locked deeply in my pockets,
And this! Some fear? Have I some apprehension?
I have forgot the walk I did take back;
Here is the gate, the door, and now it seems
My time for doubt and question must give way
To the little big role I am to play.

We breakfast and are welcomed to this place,
I will not lose that time we shared that day,
Each face betraying an eager lust to learn
From those above, enviously older.
Had they ever been afraid as we?
That morning left a strange silence in all,

It was fear that made our tongues lie still:
We all knew that our dread, like Autumn leaves,
Was falling quickly down away from us.
In happiness we meet those we'll replace:
To learn their job and learn to keep good pace.

So many times have I here been before,
Yet ne'er would I dare say I'd known this role:
So close am I to my ambition,
And yet, with some distance I do accept
The limitations of my selfishness.
I am now there, that place I will soon know:
To meet new friends and learn my part in th'show.

I can, of all my thoughts that I had lost,
(Those stolen from that moment I looked 'round),
Recall with such a clarity those scenes:
Surveying the grounds I would soon take as mine
To play my part under the team I join
Am I to think I may soon have the skills:
To grapple with the field that I survey?
I stand armed only with my past at hand,
Where shall I find that which my fate commands?

Of all colleagues of life I saw that day
I'll not forget one lady who'd lost more
Than we'd ever, God willing, ever know.
A pad and pen were her lone chance to speak:
Disease had tricked her out of word of mouth
And from the chance of life that she'd develop'd.
And she thus, robbed of dignity, did lay:
Unable to any spoken word say.

Her face e'er sad, was graced with jewels:
Her aged eyes as bright as mountain snow –
Life sapphires faceted with trials o'life.
Her strength is only matched by her weakness;
As an icicle: white and colourless.
Her dignity is lost from her I note
But for her cause can we no time devote.

The seasons alter, Spring again for my fears,
Sans sound she speaks: answers all that is asked,
And then, with little chance for a warning,
She writes more words that steal the sounds around,
So we stood, poignant as though monks at prayer,
And all our silence does is suffering bear.

So then that night do I my day recall:
It was not chance that I had lost that morn'
For 'twas a lectured second half of day,
Divorcing me from thoughts she did display.

So gently do I wipe away a tear,
Embrace, I will those values I hold dear.
In just that day had I so much not learned?
'Though not so much about my job as me:
E'en now that situation does me try;
Today's my Birthday,
The day that she wished to die.

Relationships

Introduction

Students learn a great deal during their shadowing by engaging in relationships either as participants or witnesses. Situations with patients and colleagues alike offer a means of exploring the sorts of relationships students will encounter in practice. Reading students' reflections on these relationships enables us to view quite profound and sometimes enlightening experiences that students observed. The formation of relationships in this context is crucial as a means of learning in practice.

Young doctors at the beginning of their careers are seeking to learn the shared values of the community of practice they are about to enter. This community of practice includes the entire healthcare team as well as the patients they are there for. The healthcare team's shared values are demonstrated in many ways and are particularly visible in specific encounters between professionals as well as between professionals and patients. Students identify professional norms of behaviour as they witness experienced professionals in practice.

These accounts remind us that students enter practice with optimism and positive established values which enable them to make effective critical judgements about what they perceive as good practice and those circumstances that are not in accord with their principles. They enter practice with a strong moral sense that has not been eroded by the hurly burly of their training or the healthcare system. Their descriptions of the relationships they encounter make allowances for the difficulties of practice they come across and remind us that students have much to offer the healthcare teams they are about to join.

Is it worth the bother?

When I embarked upon my two weeks of house officer shadowing, I was sure that I would not be capable of doing the job. On my first morning my confidence was boosted by being able to take blood when the nurses and the patient himself assured me that I wouldn't be able to do it. On the second day, feelings of despondency returned when I was asked by concerned nurses to see a patient with an erratic pulse who was looking pale and clammy. Unable to find my PRHO I went to the patient, feeling sure I would be no use at all. I was relieved to bump into my registrar on the way to the ward, but on arrival I found that he was relying on me to interpret the ECG. Having done this, I assessed the patient and now felt confident in my ability to be a doctor. By the end of the third day I had concluded that anybody could do the job. I was disappointed to think that six years ago I had chosen medicine as an exciting and challenging career, when in fact I would be spending at least the first three months wearily filling out hundreds of yellow and purple forms. By the end of the fourth day I was almost willing patients to develop erratic pulses.

I have decided to reflect upon the role of the PRHO in the management of one particular patient that I encountered during shadowing. He was one of only two men who were inpatients for the entire two-week duration and he had a big impact on me. He was known to have prostate cancer and was an elective admission for a radical prostatectomy.

I was taking notes during a busy ward round when he attracted my attention and told me that he was very sorry, but he had to go. He dashed off, leaving me worried as he was the next patient to be seen by the surgeons. I felt sure they would be annoyed to be held up, and in addition I was concerned that I had missed something important that I was supposed to be writing in the notes.

When we reached the patient's bed I timidly reported what the patient had said. There was some confusion, followed by the consultant checking his watch. Fortunately, the patient reappeared just at this moment. He apologised repeatedly for having kept us waiting and explained that he had been suffering from faecal incontinence since the night before. This was the first of many times in just two weeks that I was struck by just how undignified it was to be a hospital patient and I felt very sorry for this man, especially as every patient in the bay could overhear the conversation. The surgeon gently suggested that the cancer may have spread to the rectum and carried out a rectal examination. At the end of the ward round, the PRHO made a point of going back to see him to reassure him that he had not kept us waiting and empathised with him about how difficult the incontinence must be. The patient was very shocked to think that the cancer may have spread and could not understand the concept of prostate cancer spreading to the rectum. The PRHO drew a diagram to explain and subsequently the patient, although still shaken, appeared considerably less confused.

After some negotiation with the radiology department, a CT scan was performed. This confirmed that the cancer had indeed spread extensively and was now inoperable. The following morning the surgeon communicated the results to the patient and suggested that a colostomy might relieve his symptoms. The patient was visibly very upset, but continued to apologise for being so much trouble and to thank everybody for all their time and care. I found this very moving and I was close to tears because he was such a lovely unassuming man. It occurred to me that my own father would behave in a very similar way if he was in the same position. As the ward round moved on, he singled out the house officer and whispered that he had not understood what the surgeon had meant about a colostomy. The PRHO assured him that she would return later.

When we returned we explained that a colostomy would require further surgery. He was very emotional and asked whether it was worth the bother – after all, he probably didn't 'have long left'. The PRHO did not pretend to know the answers, but explained how the colostomy would work and that he would no longer have to worry about rushing to the toilet or soiling himself. She made it clear that she was not in any hurry to leave and soon the patient was confiding in her that he was very frightened and had been thinking about his death a great deal. In addition he was worried that he would not be able to cope at home on his own. The PRHO was very calm and reassuring. Immediately the patient said that it helped a tremendous amount just to talk to somebody and that our making time to see him meant a great deal to him. The PRHO gently suggested that she could make a referral to the palliative care team, explaining that this did not mean that death was imminent, but that it was a good idea to get all the support that was available.

We made a referral to the palliative care team, and telephoned and wrote a referral note to the general surgeons, asking for their opinion regarding a colostomy. We spoke to his nurses, who were also very concerned about him and had organised for him to see the chaplain and a specialist oncology nurse. When I finished my attachment he was being prepared for surgery.

Witnessing the care of this patient over two weeks has illustrated a number of important points. The PRHO has a very important role in communicating with many different people. Of prime importance is communication with the patient – explaining anything which is unclear and delivering bad news and test results in an appropriate way. The other members of her team were often busy in theatre and it fell on her to be a constant figure on the ward that the patient recognised as someone that he could talk to. In this case the PRHO also had to discuss and negotiate the patient's care with her own team, the general surgeons, the nurses, the palliative care team and the radiology department.

I realised that although much of the job is secretarial, some patients require a great deal more attention and thought. It is these patients who make the job worthwhile and interesting. I am determined that I too will be an approachable house officer that patients can talk to and trust to give them correct information. It is essential to have good communication skills – including the ability to listen to the patient without hurrying them. The value of sitting in silence while the patient gathered his thoughts and formulated questions was demonstrated several times. I thoroughly look forward to beginning my job in August – yellow forms and all!

The doctor–patient relationship

Following my PRHO shadowing, my reflections have turned most often to that valuable health resource; the doctor–patient relationship. To empathise, to form that affinity with patients – this was my primary motivation for becoming a doctor in the beginning! I suppose I assumed maintaining this position would become an integral part of my personality – instinct as opposed to a conscious process. I didn't consider myself naïve. I have two grandparents who have unfortunately developed dementia, and I recognised in them some of the challenges I might face as their personalities fragmented and they became aggressive and fearful facing this disintegration.

Now, as I contemplate the fact that in August, I will *actually* be a doctor (gulp!), I do feel there is a part of me that sends out antennae, and helps me sense my way when communicating with every patient. To an extent, I was right – I am becoming a communication machine! However, shadowing has enforced two more realisations – first, that the more confident I become at establishing this rapport, the more discordantly it seems to be rebuffed. And, second, that sometimes this rapport can hurt if it's not limited. To illustrate this, I have two patients I would like to discuss.

The first patient had been admitted 12 days before I arrived with severe pneumonia and confusion. The confusion had resolved, although she retained a slight underlying dementia, and had little insight into her condition. Unfortunately, my first impression of her was that she was a most unpleasant, cantankerous lady. However, as hospital frequently does not display people to their best advantage, as they are often worried, frightened, and just plain ill, I tried to circumvent that first impression, and continue treating her with the respect and warmth I hope someone treating my own cantankerous grandmother might display. I've found in the past that squeezing out a modicum of extra sympathy and understanding allows me to find something likeable in all my patients. Not so this poor lady. Maybe it was that the ward was closed due to Norwalk virus, so we had fewer patients than normal. Maybe it was being mentally more involved as a team member. And maybe she really was a particularly difficult lady but, whatever it was, I really couldn't like her. I felt that handling the doctor–patient relationship with no liking on my part to drive it was like travelling downhill in a car with the engine off – it goes, but feels wrong. I felt guilty; as if I wasn't doing my job properly.

This all sounds rather negative, but actually this is a *positive* reflection. I never learned to *like* this lady, and I don't think anyone else did either, judging by the general level of grumbling! However, every day, some or all of the team would do the round and, every day, she would regale us with abuse – we were keeping her prisoner here, we didn't know our jobs, she had never been ill anyway, etc. And, every day, someone would give her a little extra time and space, and explain the current and past situation to her with impeccable kindliness and respect, trying to maximise her level of understanding and mitigate what fear she might be feeling. I saw everybody on the team behave in this way, from the consultant to the PRHO, and suddenly realised that I was doing it too. I don't feel her care was compromised in any way, despite what the underlying emotions of the team might have been, unless there really is some mythical healing connection between healer and patient – in which case, she appeared to be subsisting and recovering fairly well on a less ethereal plane.

The next case involved Mr and Mrs D. Mr D was a 75-year-old gentleman who presented to A&E with a dense stroke. My PRHO and I were on call, and we decided I should see Mr D, in the role of the house officer. Mr D was unconscious and virtually unresponsive when I arrived to see him, so I obtained a history from his wife. Mrs D was one of the most delightful people I've ever been privileged to meet, and was trying hard to hide the deep distress she was feeling. Obtaining a rapport with her was exceptionally easy, as I was able to fetch her the first cup of tea she'd had for four hours. She told me that Mr D had been doing chores in the garden, she wandered out to see where he had got to, and found him collapsed and unresponsive. It was unexpected – he had mild early Alzheimer's but was otherwise well. She was outwardly cheerful and calm, and even joked a little bit, yet often her hands would clutch at the warmth of the paper cup, and her eyes fix on a point somewhere over my shoulder, and contract as if contemplating something terrible, before flying back to the detached clinical environment of the hospital. She would then revert to cheerful mode. I respected that this was probably her coping mechanism, and responded accordingly.

Eventually, the A&E SHO and I had to break the news to Mrs D which she had already guessed, that her husband would probably not recover, and she did eventually allow herself to cry, apologising, as if protecting us from her distress was more important than her entitlement to express it.

The whole event was handled very well – everyone was sympathetic and caring. Several people commented on how lovely Mrs D was, but, as for the other patient I have described, their personal feelings did not overwhelm professional management – mine nearly did. When Mrs D started to cry, my eyes and throat starting burning, and I was profoundly grateful that I didn't have to speak.

When the SHO broke the bad news, she emphasised that she was stressing a worst case scenario, so staggering the shock. Mrs D was being collected by neighbours; her sons were travelling down, but would not arrive for some hours. As she waited for them, I re-emphasised that it was too early to know what would happen for sure. In retrospect, I wonder if that was the right thing to do (he died two days later) – perhaps a little hope would be a boon, as she waited alone in her newly empty house, at least until her sons arrived and she had support. Or was I offering reassurance for myself as well as Mrs D? I was definitely too emotionally involved, although at least I managed to hide it, and maintain a professional image. I felt a surge of quite unreasonable anger when people said the stroke could in ways 'have been a blessing', as Mr D's Alzheimer's would have torn through both their lives eventually. The likely truth behind that rather glib phrase had never seemed more overshadowed by the anguish of the here and now. I found myself thinking what a cold, inhuman place the department must seem to a patient, how little it engendered the right feelings to say goodbye to someone.

I'll never survive as a doctor if I constantly allow myself to become overwhelmed in what is essentially someone else's heartbreak. On the other hand, some emotional involvement seems vital to stay human. Mrs D made me feel vulnerable, and she has probably helped me learn what it takes to achieve that equilibrium.

In both these cases the emotional background behind the doctor–patient relationship differed from the norm, yet both cases received the same level of commitment – neither was compromised or given unfair advantage as a result. Everyone played out their roles and responsibilities as expected and good communication benefited both patients. Perhaps this is where communication 'skills' really come in – to allow health professionals to cope when such situations arise.

I still feel communication is a valuable resource, and feel quite confident. I still feel a lot of it is instinctive. Yet perhaps the greater involvement, new role and different experiences of communicating during shadowing has really made me realise that, like every other clinical skill, I will need to keep honing this skill as a continuous learning process.

Please grant that I never become disillusioned, embittered or, worse, just lose interest.

Striving for holistic care

I had always looked forward to our shadowing course with some trepidation. The prospect of gaining first-hand experience of what life will be like beyond the sheltered environment of medical school was at the same time exciting and terrifying. The prospect of shouldering grave responsibility for real people's lives with what still feels like very rudimentary medical knowledge is scary and I was all too aware that this was the first time that it would be real. In short, it required growing up.

I approached the ward on Tuesday morning with mixed feelings. This was the first time I could legitimately feel needed and not adopt the perennially apologetic medical student role for merely being alive. I repeated my now familiar mantra of the preceding weeks – be confident, be professional and believe you can do this. It sounds vaguely ridiculous but was absolutely necessary.

The ward was lovely. It comprised 16 beds for elderly ladies, the majority awaiting social care packages and most of whom also had some degree of dementia. Working there absolutely required the holistic approach to healthcare we are encouraged to wheel out at every available opportunity to demonstrate our ability to look after the 'whole patient'. However, the reality on this ward was that many of the patients were far more concerned that they didn't feel able to cope at home or that the dog was being looked after than whether they had a pansystolic murmur or slightly low sodium. In order to establish any kind of therapeutic relationship with these patients it was essential to recognise these very important needs.

All the staff were very welcoming. I was given a whistle-stop tour of the ward and introduced to the patients and staff. I was provided with the various codes for the staff-room door and shown the location of the myriad forms and telephone numbers in the ward office which I promptly forgot. The house officer supplied me with a list of the patients and comprehensive description of the various ailments, test results, pending investigations and home situation. He then provided me with another list of the jobs for the day and a guide as to where to find free lunch every day of the week. Phew! I was rather overwhelmed. I fear I may not have made the sparkling impression I had intended in my mantra. Instead I spent the rest of the day asking all the same questions we had discussed earlier. However, I also had the opportunity to meet some of the patients and found myself far more able to remember the interminable lists of clinical details recorded on the patient list when I could put a face to the name. I left exhausted and determined to do better on Wednesday.

I arrived the following morning to find the house officer and SHO deep in conversation over a set of blood results. It transpired that a lady admitted with severe leg ulcers had become increasingly drowsy overnight and that her renal function was deteriorating rather unexpectedly. This baffled the medical team as they could find no obvious precipitant. We watched her closely for the rest of the day and to our disappointment she continued declining rapidly. By late afternoon when her daughter came to visit she had become delirious and was screaming in pain, begging for someone to relieve her misery. We explained as best we could what we thought had happened and that, while we were intending to continue active treatment, given her various co-morbidities we were not optimistic about a good recovery.

This scenario was all too familiar to me. I could genuinely empathise with the bleak, desperate and frightened expression on her daughter's face. Last year my grandmother developed sepsis following a bowel perforation and spent a protracted period in intensive care following surgery. Four years' clinical experience could not prepare me for my first visit to the intensive care unit and seeing my own grandmother as 'the patient'; for the first time a familiar, beloved face, all too obviously suffering. I also understood her daughter's struggle to understand what was going on, intellectually able to comprehend but frightened and being in an alien environment with no familiar points of reference, particularly any coherent response from her mother. I had witnessed similar consultations on numerous occasions previously but now that I really understood and could provide a context it was an altogether more difficult experience.

The next day I was not surprised but nevertheless disappointed to discover that there had been no improvement in the lady's condition. Her daughter arrived soon after I did; desperately trying to remain composed, smiling and greeting everyone and enquiring politely as to any recent changes. Our ward round eventually reached them and we had a frank discussion with the daughter as to what her mother would have wanted. She explained that her mother had been suffering dreadfully for years from her leg ulcers and would not want any intervention. She bravely maintained her composure until she described her mother's intolerance of people who were 'precious about death' and her own extraordinarily philosophical and somewhat irreverent approach. Then her daughter broke down, brittle tears that could not be controlled. 'It's just I know what she's like normally,' she explained. 'She would hate this.' We all agreed to withdraw active treatment and to keep her as comfortable as possible.

Over the following days we watched the inexorable decline in her renal function and clinical condition. Fortunately we managed to control her pain more successfully and she spent most days sleeping peacefully. During this time her daughter kept an almost constant vigil at her bedside, always arriving with a newspaper but invariably leaving it unread, preferring instead to spend her visits watching her mother's face and talking to her quietly. We all awaited her demise.

I was therefore astounded to arrive on the ward on Monday to discover that the most recent blood tests showed that her renal function had normalised. I approached her bed to see for myself her observations chart and miraculous improvement in urine output and was even more surprised to be greeted by a weary smile. 'I do apologise if I caused any trouble,' she said. We had a long conversation about her recent illness while I tried to alleviate her fears that she had disrupted the entire ward screaming. I gave her a glass of water and she drank greedily. When she had drained the last drop she grinned toothily at me. 'Thanks,' she said. 'You're an angel.'

For the rest of the day the noise in the ward was punctuated not by the sound of screaming but instead by loud and enthusiastic apologies for causing trouble and lengthy exposition as to the nature of health and illness. We were delighted. Her daughter arrived shortly after her mother had been washed and she found her surveying the ward, hair freshly brushed and beautifully presented in her bed jacket, quite unrecognisable from recent days.

I have the dubious privilege of having been on both sides. I understand the various pressures on junior doctors and that it can be frustrating if a plan of management is changed halfway through. I have witnessed how difficult it can be to accommodate the preferences and needs of families in patient care. I realise how extraordinarily difficult it can be to provide appropriate analgesia when apparently all the options have been tested and none seems to be adequate. I also understand that on occasions time pressures mean that it can be difficult to spend as much time as we would like with our patients. However, I also understand how frightening and bewildering it can be to be 'the rellies' when it seems that no one will explain what is going on. I have experienced fractious doctors becoming aggressive when they perceive that their care is being challenged or questioned. I understand as a 'rellie' how frustrating it can be when someone close to you, who is at their most vulnerable, is suffering and no one appears to be listening or trying to relieve that suffering.

It required very little time or extra effort to talk to the lady's daughter and to try to understand what she thought was best for her mother. I could act as their advocate and communicate their feelings to the rest of the team. I tried to listen when her daughter was concerned about her pain and we explored different analgesic options. I could also celebrate with the daughter when her mother so surprisingly improved.

Ideally when I start work I will meet the requirements of my mantra. I will sparkle and become renowned through the hospital as a competent and brilliant doctor. I will remember where to find all the forms and never forget to label blood bottles. Of course I will never need to ask my SHO to insert a difficult venflon because I can't find a vein. However, increasingly I come to realise that, while these skills are important, we must not lose sight of our other responsibilities.

As doctors we have the privilege of being able to provide care for people and their families with unique personalities, experiences, preconceptions, priorities and expectations. Sometimes both patient and relative will be suspicious, difficult or deeply unappreciative of the efforts being made for them or their relative. Invariably however these people are also suffering. I hope that I will appreciate this privilege and be able to alleviate some of their suffering without resenting their questions and concerns. Idealistic? Maybe. Realistic? Ultimately yes. Effective in patient care? Definitely. As clinicians we will inevitably know more about the clinical circumstances of a patient than a relative but the relative will know more about the patient as a person. All are required to contribute (and to have a voice) if the treatment of a patient is to be genuinely holistic.

Can I do anything to help?

A fortnight in hospital medicine for some is chance to gain vital extra moments of learning experience; for others who yearn to be waged, it offers time to see if it really is all worth it; for those who want only that their time be no longer governed by guilt and regret, it offers a valid excuse to get away from textbooks; and for some people in hospital medicine it's two weeks of emotional torture. We can so easily forget the patients.

'Today's just going to be a business round,' says my consultant 'Oh,' says I, who, feeling particularly eloquent, tried in one word to express the deep sinking feeling I commonly feel as I know the rest of my morning will be spent running after stethoscoped office clerks. One could imagine, in the style of the city-bound genre so often portrayed on hospital ward rounds, that employee star-ranked business ethics may become key to ward work. Patients would be scored highly for smiling at their consultants, allowing the juniors to scribble 'Obs stable – plan: home soon', for enthusiastically taking on the patient role, and for being pleasant and courteous to all those gifted with the pleasure of their company during their hospital stay. Those with low scores may have to remain in hospital for more 'training' while those with high scores will be allowed to graduate back into society.

Mrs C is almost a five-star patient in her hospital ward. This 84-year-old lady has done well since her admission. She was fully investigated and treated for her urinary tract infection. She now is stable and medically fit for discharge. But she has not been allowed to 'graduate' because she suffers from dementia, and repetitively shouts the same short indistinguishable four-syllable phrase during the night from her bed, keeping other patients awake.

'How's Mrs C today?' says the consultant. 'No change,' says the PRHO, 'awaiting social work review.' She looks at the consultant with fear in her eyes. No smiles. 'Good then … Next patient.'

Mrs C has been in hospital for several months now as her husband is unable to care for her and an EMI is the only option for her long-term care. I have seen many patients remain in hospital while in this apparent state of 'well-being'. At first I thought only of my regular frustration at seeing yet another 'bed-blocking' elderly patient, desperately in need of a well-funded and effectively resourced social care system. But then, in the middle of my second week when I was shadowing my PRHO's 'second-on-call' duties, I was called to Mrs C's side by frustrated nurses, who were unable to bring calm to their ward and extinguish the lights as normal at 11 pm. Mrs C was chanting her familiar four-syllable phrase: 'on the toilet', 'but don't tell it' – nobody was quite sure. I knelt by Mrs C's bed and looked into her eyes. Quietly I began to address the reason for her shouting, with questions: 'What's the matter? Can I do anything to help?' And her only response was to look at me and begin to cry ... but the shouting had stopped. I was slightly taken aback by this change of behaviour and obvious sign of distress, in someone who had seemed to me to be such a distant mind. I waited a few seconds before acknowledging that, although afflicted by a socially debilitating condition, Mrs C was a real person, and must be responding as any 'normal' person would, in distress. My questions turned to reassuring statements: 'You are safe here. The people you see around you will look after you. Try resting your head back and closing your eyes.'

And sure enough after no more than two or three minutes, Mrs C was asleep, and the ward could finally begin its nocturnal routine.

Something needs to be done NOW!

The incident that I have chosen for this reflective account occurred during a night on call with the PRHO that I was shadowing. This shift was to involve covering all the medical wards in the hospital and as such had the potential to be very busy. The reason I chose to write about this particular night was that first it did indeed turn out to be rather busy but also it probably highlighted and illustrated much of what a soon-to-be-qualified medical student may fear about the 'dreaded night shifts'. The feeling of being alone in dealing with difficult clinical situations, difficult patients and dare I say it insistent nurses expecting decisions made and action taken – NOW!

The night began fairly calmly and it seemed at this point that it may well drag on pretty slowly; I was already beginning to feel sleepy. However, things were soon to become significantly more challenging. The next call came asking us to come and re-site a cannula in a patient who had taken hers out and was being disruptive on the ward. The patient turned out to be a young woman suffering from end-stage liver failure due to alcohol abuse. She was oozing blood from her gums, was vomiting up large amounts of blood and had blood dripping out of her arm due to the ripped out cannula. She was stomping up and down the ward shouting and wailing with a trail of nurses behind her trying to keep her away from the other patients. The nurse in charge, quite understandably, was insistent that we needed to do something about her now. However, the patient was confused, upset and fairly out of control. By this time the porters had arrived to physically control the lady if needed and the nurse in charge was becoming increasingly insistent that action was needed now. On one side of us the ward was in disarray as the lady continued to rush around the ward, bleeding and shouting; on the other side was the nurse in charge insisting that we sedate the lady now. The nurse was asking for haloperidol to be administered immediately; the PRHO had never prescribed haloperidol before and wasn't sure how much to give. Eventually in the face of much insistence from the nurses and the patient in the background causing bedlam, the maximum dose of 10 mg of haloperidol was given and not surprisingly the lady went out like a light not soon after!

For me this incident illustrated a number of important aspects of the work of the F1 doctor and also picked up on a number of themes from the shadowing course. The incident described was one in which the PRHO was not sure how to act or what to do, and personally the situation was quite a scary one, particularly when thinking that in a few months this could be me asked to make this decision.

The incident, rather abruptly, illustrated the roles and responsibilities of the PRHO on call in all too graphic a way. The PRHO was the doctor called to make a decision about a patient's treatment there and then and to do something about it. This is a rather different and daunting situation to that of being a medical student where decisions and action are very rarely called for in such a crucial way. This for me was the first time I had witnessed a fairly junior doctor having to make such a decision without any more senior input or assistance. To a more experienced doctor the decision may not have seemed so daunting, but to me, and I think the PRHO also, administering a powerful antipsychotic drug to a seriously ill lady was a fairly big deal!

In addition the incident also made me reflect on the clinical skills required by the F1 doctor. Being on call for the whole hospital for the night brought home to me just how much medical knowledge one needs to have to be able confidently to deal with the variety of situations that rear their head in the middle of the night. In this situation I was strangely encouraged by the way the PRHO didn't have all the answers and was madly thumbing through the BNF for inspiration. It made me realise that I didn't have to know everything and that even though the PRHO didn't know what to do at first the patient didn't come to any harm and the situation was resolved.

Lastly this situation also highlighted the importance of communication skills and the interprofessional team in which we work. This was a good example of the tensions between different parts of the team and their roles; in this case the nurses endeavouring to protect the integrity of the ward and the comfort of the other patients and the doctor trying to decide on what medically was the best option for the patient given her co-morbidities. In situations such as this one it is not only the patient that we are managing but also our relationships with other team members and how well we do this is dependent on our communication skills.

Situations requiring quick but reasoned decisions require a certain degree of knowledge but in addition a considerable confidence in being able to make those important decisions; the transition from student to doctor involves a huge change in roles and as such a change in the way that other staff interact with you and what they expect from you. This is certainly an area that I am looking forward to developing.

An apology

Our shadowing fortnight is there to enable us to prepare for what is the next major step in our lives. It serves as a chance to familiarise ourselves with what is to come once medical school and graduation are behind us. Yet I don't think that any amount of formal preparation will ever prepare the final year medical student for what is perhaps the steepest learning curve he or she will ever have to face. My shadowing experience was a mere taster of that curve and if anything it made me realise paradoxically how much knowledge and understanding I have acquired over the last five years, and yet how very little that seems to amount to when faced with the reality of being a PRHO.

It is strange how very differently I found myself thinking and feeling as I walked onto what was to become 'my ward' and met the staff whom I was soon to join as part of their team. A 'real' part with 'real' responsibility, so exciting and yet extremely daunting. It was fascinating to see the difference in attitude towards me, as a student in a different guise. It suddenly became apparent when I was introduced as 'your new PRHO' that my opinion mattered and I, despite being the same student I had been in the lecture theatre the day before, was now both more trusted and respected. It was a wonderful feeling!

I gained so much during the fortnight that selecting one event to reflect upon is an almost impossible task. However, there was one particular lesson I don't think I will ever forget for both good and bad reasons.

The days of the doctor being 'God and Master' over both patients and the health professional team are long gone. Throughout our course the value of good communication with both patients and colleagues has been emphasised and re-emphasised to us. In everything we do we are taught to approach medicine from the patient's point of view and as part of a multidisciplinary team. It was therefore interesting and enlightening to see the difficulties we will all face at putting some of this philosophy into practice and it made me realise that although we all feel we will never forget our patient-centred dictum we are still as fallible as the next person.

It was a busy Tuesday morning post-take ward round. As ever there were too many patients and too little time and the consultant was not in good humour. As is often the case this mood seemed to have rubbed off onto his team and the group of disgruntled doctors around the bedside of an elderly gentleman must have seemed an unhappy and unapproachable bunch. What was to evolve over the next 10 minutes will stay with me for the duration of my career as it made me truly appreciate the power of apology.

The patient was unwell; he was awaiting a second amputation for peripheral vascular disease. His ulcers were infected and he was in a considerable amount of pain. Several things seemed to have gone wrong. The nurses had recently dressed the patient's wounds so the consultant became angry that he could not see the ulcers. The nurse with us was young and he spoke to her patronisingly, asking her what on earth she thought she was doing bringing him to see a patient's leg ulcers when there would 'clearly be nothing to see, like this'. His tone of voice and attitude brought her to the edge of tears and standing around the patient we could all feel the tension rising. The nurse apologised, politely saying that it had not been documented that the consultant would want to see them today. He replied that he had not realised that he now had to run every decision past the junior nursing staff and asked her to go and get someone who 'had a clue what was going on'. He then turned to the senior house officer and berated him for not ensuring that 'his PRHO' documented what he said, adding that 'it is not as if they have anything else to do these days'. The PRHO was standing beside him and he did not look at her once. The consultant then finally turned to the patient and asked him how he was. 'Appalled,' the patient answered. 'Never in my 86 years have I heard a caring young lady spoken to in such a way. You are a very nice man Mr X, you have given me the best care and treatment I could wish for, but don't ever forget who it is who looks after us once you have wielded your knife.'

The consultant looked abashed and I half-expected him to dismiss the patient and leave but he did not. He sat down on the bed, apologised to the patient for having the disagreement across his bed, agreed that, yes, the patient was right and said that he would also apologise to the nurse involved. He then conducted his consultation in a friendly and caring manner. After the ward round he apologised to the nurse involved and then to all of us, saying that it was no excuse but that he had been having a bad morning. He added that we must never forget to listen to our patients! It turned out he had had some bad news the previous evening but had insisted on coming to work.

I had never heard a consultant apologise in this way before and I respected him greatly for admitting his mistake. The incident served to remind me of the pressures that we put ourselves under and it was refreshing and reassuring to see that even the most senior doctors are vulnerable to the outside pressures of life and are not 'superhuman' and able to completely separate work and home life.

It also taught me the immense importance of mutual respect within the medical team and the power of admitting we are wrong and simply saying sorry. Despite what we are taught as students, in the real world, on a day-to-day basis with the stresses and frustrations imposed upon us, it can be difficult not to get angry and lay blame when things don't get done.

In conclusion I found the shadowing fortnight immensely important and enjoyable. I think I am far from ready for the job I am about to do, but I certainly feel more prepared than I did, not in terms of knowledge about disease and management but more in relation to people, both those I will be working for and those I will have the privilege of caring for. I am excited about the prospect of what August holds for me and feel that now when it comes to sink or swim I have got a fighting chance to make it to the other side.

Two patients with chest pain

I really enjoyed my shadowing weeks. It felt great to be introduced to a firm as the next house officer and not just another pesky medical student. The experience not only gave me confidence that I will manage the job in August but it also gave me a boost to my revision. The knowledge I had was suddenly relevant and useful in day-to-day decisions and it made me eager to learn more. Working in a team was also fun since I have spent much of my time on the wards as a student alone. I like having other people relying on what I do and the pressure of a time limit followed by the satisfaction of completing the tasks assigned to me. I have chosen two situations on which to reflect.

In all our breaking bad news sessions the news is usually cancer and either telling the patient they have cancer for the first time or that their treatment options are palliative. Very rarely does the scenario involve respiratory disease, heart disease or stroke. It is easy to forget that common diseases and diagnoses are still shocking for the person experiencing them for the first time. The diagnosis might seem so obvious to the doctors they assume the patient is up to speed with developments and is already fully aware of their diagnosis. Patients with diseases that get a lot of publicity, for example heart disease, are often very well informed or have family members who have dealt with a similar experience. However, for some the news is devastating and breaking this news should be done as sympathetically as if the diagnosis was cancer.

On a ward round a patient asked what exactly had happened to him. He was not sure what his chest pain meant or why he was suddenly put on a long list of tablets when he previously had taken nothing but a couple of paracetamol for the occasional headache. When the consultant explained that he had had a heart attack he was really very surprised and anxious. He was unsure how serious this was and what implications it had for his job as a carpenter. I was not expecting him to be so shocked by the diagnosis or anxious about the future. Most patients are aware they are having a heart attack and so by the time they are on the ward awaiting an angiogram they have read all the leaflets several times and asked many questions. It reinforced the importance of checking what the patient understands has happened so far, before assuming they are aware of what has happened to them at each step. Most people would rather not have to take a handful of tablets every morning and adjusting to this is difficult. Tablets make them feel like someone with an illness and they don't want to be reminded every day of their increased risk of a heart attack.

The next learning point was from a post-take handover early one morning (it's not just surgeons who start at 8 am!). The SHO presented a patient who had experienced chest pain the previous day. In the past medical history he mentioned her problems with vertigo and dizziness, which had been thoroughly investigated by the ENT doctors but no cause had been found. The consultant went to see her and told her it was inappropriate to investigate her chest pain in the usual way in light of her undiagnosed vertigo and dizziness. He felt she was a patient for the ENT doctors. I was most upset by his complete lack of interest in any patient without pure heart disease. She was not a complicated patient other than her idiopathic vertigo and deserved the same treatment and investigations as any other cardiac patient. The patient looked horrified as the consultant dismissed her symptoms of chest pain and swept away in a flurry of unsigned exercise tolerance test, angiogram and echocardiogram request forms.

I call this the danger of specialisation. Some doctors seem to have a mortal fear or overpowering disinterest in a patient with a concurrent disease for which they have no knowledge or experience. However, this patient is still a patient with chest pain regardless of how dizzy our visit left her! What I learned from this is that presenting is a very powerful tool. You hold the important information for that patient and how they are subsequently treated can depend on your ability to present their history. Obviously no facts should be omitted but the emphasis can be subtly altered. As the admitting house officer it is important not to let your patient down in this act of transferring information.

The two key issues I have reflected on are simple but important. The first is to never forget the impact of a diagnosis on the life of a patient. All issues surrounding breaking news to patients should follow the same principles learned in palliative care. This is to take the patient on a journey to the discovery of the current situation regarding their health. This journey is best started from the level of understanding the patient has of their current diagnosis or prognosis. It is best to catch a train from a platform than leaping for it as it zooms past James Bond style, which is likely to result in injury! Ask before speaking will be my motto.

The second issue highlighted how important the role of a PRHO is for every patient you clerk. Despite being at the bottom of the ladder we have a great influence over the care our patients receive. I look forward to rising to this responsibility.

Working for Dr X

The incident I have decided to write about is a post-take ward round with one of the consultants in general medicine. To preserve anonymity I shall call her Dr X. I chose this 'incident' because her behaviour draws out many issues, some of which are reflected as 'vertical themes' in the medical course – for example ethics, communication skills and radiology. It is important to stress that there was no single event prompting me to write this report – I simply felt that, in general, this ward round highlighted some important issues.

Post-take ward rounds begin at 8 am. As a junior (or a student) it is advisable to get there about 10 minutes earlier – that way it is possible to draw up a list of patients admitted on the take; these lists often include details like hospital number and presenting complaint. I arrived and introduced myself to one member of the nursing staff. 'Ahh, a medical student,' she said, 'you'll be going around with Dr X – good luck …' She rolled her eyes and hurried away. As is so often the way in hospital, another member of staff heard part of the conversation and asked for confirmation: 'Is it Dr X this morning?' 'Yes,' I answered. The nurse's shoulders sagged visibly.

In my previous years at medical school these kind of responses would have produced a wide-eyed adrenaline rush of anxiety. What if I get the answers wrong/look stupid? What if she shouts at me?

But that morning I wasn't worried. I now tend to laugh when confronted with erratic, twitchy seniors. Maybe it's experience. Maybe it's cynicism. I laugh at the crazy consultant, at myself, at THE SYSTEM and its institutional stupidity. I don't laugh out loud though. Maybe it's hysteria. Anyway, that morning I wasn't worried. Besides, I knew I had a reflective account to write. This could be material!

So Dr X arrives in a bustle of forceful activity. A tired, forlorn-looking SHO mentions that 30 patients were admitted last night. The tone in his voice and bags under his eyes betray his thought – 'I was up all night, and I still have 30 patients to get through so please, PLEASE Dr X can we get through it as quickly as possible?' 'So what,' snaps Dr X, already feeling she is being rushed, 'this is nothing unusual, we've been having heavy takes recently.' With that she sweeps off. We (house officer, SHO, nurse) gather ourselves around her and swoop down to the first patient.

We sweep and swoop all morning, and until 1.30 in the afternoon. The ward round still hasn't finished but I have scheduled teaching and therefore a legitimate excuse to leave.

I have had plenty of time to think about why people don't like Dr X. She is not a rude lady, I think, but she does have difficulties communicating with other member of staff and patients. In her haste to get things done she sometimes forgets that people need a moment to absorb what they have been told or asked.

For example, one middle-aged man had been admitted with ECG changes and cardiac chest pain. He smokes 25 cigarettes a day. Dr X examines his chest and asks her first question. 'Do you want to give up smoking?' she says, one ear still engaged by her stethoscope. The man falters, umms and ahhs. 'Because if you do I can put a patch right ...' – she smartly taps his upper arm – '... here'. The patient, in pain, in an unfamiliar environment and quite likely convalescing from a heart attack, cannot recover his wits quickly enough to answer. 'I thought not,' says Dr X and turns to leave. As she reaches the end of his bed she spins on her heel to face him again, as if she had just remembered something. 'But KNOW THIS ...' Her voice takes on a prophetic quality. 'If your life was this long ...' – she holds her hands wide apart – '... YOU have made it ... this long'. Her thumb and forefinger are nearly touching, holding an imaginary grain of rice between them.

The staff have problems with her too. 'She over-investigates everybody,' says the house officer. 'The radiologists hate her,' another doctor tells me. I can see their point. Nearly every patient on the ward round was sent for an echocardiogram. To my mind over-investigation is not only a resource issue but an ethical one too. After all, if the result isn't going to change the management, should the patient be inconvenienced by the investigation in the first place? And what of appropriate patients whose echos are delayed because of unnecessary testing? It's not only echos though. 'No other consultant makes as much work for her juniors,' one of the house officers tells me.

Dr X provided me with an interesting situation to write about. There are some concluding points I would like to make.

1. Feeling like a patient. I found it interesting that it was obvious to me, right from the start, that the staff disliked Dr X, but that feeling was never communicated in an explicit way. Every bad connotation was a shrugged shoulder, a rolled eye or telling me how somebody else (e.g. the radiologists) disliked her. Is this how people act when they don't like 'the boss'? Is this behaviour limited to the ward? Probably not. Nonetheless I felt the way a patient should never (but I suspect often does) feel – that something bad was happening and nobody would tell me what it was.

2. Judgement. The purpose of this essay is not to judge Dr X but to examine the reactions of those around her (i.e. staff and patients). Perhaps she is right to order so many investigations. Perhaps the juniors will always resent someone who 'makes more work' for them. Interestingly, one patient I spoke to had warmed to her despite her brusque manner. 'I feel as if she's very thorough ... doing everything she can.'

3. Reflection. Reflection is holding a mirror to the world. In this case the mirror (i.e. me) has been beaten into shape by nearly five years of medical training. Perhaps somebody without that training would have seen a completely different ward round, and highlighted different issues. Perhaps someone with even more training (e.g. Dr X) would see different issues again. Reflection is a basic human quality and an activity in which we all participate.

4. Working for Dr X next year. Since this was my shadowing week, how do I feel about working for Dr X next year? The answer is I won't be. She moves to a different hospital at the end of the month!

Will it kill me?

'Is this serious?'
'Um … Yes.'
'Gosh. Very serious?'
'Yes, it probably is.'
'Will it kill me?'
'Well, yes it will. Anyway, would it be all right if I talked through your bronchoscopy this afternoon with some nurses that I'm training?'

I was on a ward round with the respiratory firm when I listened to the above conversation between the consultant and a 60-year-old anxious patient who had been admitted with a cough, a suspicious shadow on her chest x-ray and a past medical history of breast cancer. I had met her for the first time a few hours previously when I cannulated her and we had a brief chat. As soon as she had given her consent for the training afternoon, the curtains were whisked back and the whole firm left her all alone with this devastating new information while they carried on their ward round.

I was horrified and found that I was unable to follow the rest of the firm out. I had been with the firm earlier when they discussed her case – I had also heard the nurses talking about how anxious this patient had been since her admission. I decided that now was the time to have my first shot at the doctor's infamous role of breaking bad news. While I was on my medical placement I visited the local hospice. The palliative care physician there spent the morning with us and we all found him very inspiring. The following week he gave an excellent lecture to all the students and housemen about breaking bad news. One of the main points he made was to always be truthful with the patient and to give them hope.

The lecture stuck in my mind and I redrew the patient's curtains and sat down on her bed. She had lots of questions – some of which I was able to answer, and some of which I had to say that I did not know the answer to, but that she must remember to ask the doctor when she next saw him. Her main worry was that she was going to be left alone to deal with this unsupported and I was able to confidently reassure her that this would not be the case. Her brother arrived after 10 or 15 minutes and, when I said goodbye, she thanked me for the time that I had spent with her. I rejoined the ward round, feeling rather distanced and surreal, and later found the lady's nurse to tell her exactly what I had said to her patient.

Why was this important to me? I have written about this incident as it has frequently been on my mind. What would I have done if I had been the house officer in that situation? This poses a very relevant dilemma. Obviously, as housemen, we cannot follow the ward round in the wake of the team clearing up unfinished issues – we need to be there for the next patient. I have come to the conclusion that, if needed, we will have to limit ourselves to reassuring the patient that we will be back at the end of the ward round to answer any more questions that they have. Then, of course, we will have to make sure that we do make the time to go back.

I think that the breaking of bad news deserves particular attention because of the significance to the patient. We have all been told, and indeed know from our own experience, that when something has been done badly it will be remembered forever. Telling somebody that they have cancer is not something that we can afford to do badly.

I thought that this brief interaction was an example of horrifically poor communication skills. I do, however, realise that doctors simply do not have the time to spend hours with each of their patients answering questions, and that after breaking bad news day after day for many years, one must become desensitised to it. I do think that at the moment my fellow students and I are all reasonably good communicators and I worry that when we are tired and busy we will have less empathy for our patients. We will have to make a conscious effort to stop this from happening, and to remind ourselves of how embarrassed we sometimes felt as students watching situations like this occur.

What can I learn from this incident?

- Not to break bad news like that.
- To never lose touch with how we must appear to the patient – after all, they are why we are here in the first place.
- To learn to fulfil my role as the firm's house officer and to manage my time efficiently.
- I realise that I will often be telling patients unwanted news and that, unfortunately, I will probably also be witnessing sensitive doctor–patient interactions that are poorly handled. I must learn not to dwell for too long on upsetting incidents, but to learn from them and move on.

The incident that I have described summarises only one of the many day-to-day observations that we make and learn from. Some of these encounters are very positive and are logged to remind me to follow suit when it becomes our turn. Work shadowing was a fantastic, informative experience and a very enjoyable week.

Becoming the chain makers

The objective of this particular attachment, an experience that many would describe as fundamentally the most important and indeed most relevant two-week attachment within the fifth year medical curriculum, was to prepare us, the final year medical student, for the daunting reality of being a fully grown doctor, in the not too distant future. So, what was I, the student, expecting to gain from this experience? Was it an opportunity to become familiar with the general quirky habits and traditions of the hospital, the computer system, the form filling-in role, where the blood bottles are hidden, which nurses to befriend and who to supply with regular caffeine fixes? Or was it perhaps one final chance to reconfirm the fear and anticipation of our forthcoming role as the PRHO, already firmly rooted in each and every one of us?

On reflection, all of the above was achieved, alongside a whole lot more. The medical curriculum is itself associated with a steep learning curve and this attachment was no exception; in fact, it was perhaps the steepest curve to date, steep, information-overloaded, but, most of all, invaluable. During this short time I feel that my medical education and experiences were enhanced in ways that they have not been in the past. For the first time in five years, I was exposed to the forefront of medical care without the label of the short white coat and the stigma of the medical student. I was a peer about to embark upon a role that had a purpose and identity. I was to become a proper member of the team and was thus treated as such. On a personal level, being included enhances one's own morale; but it also aids for a better learning experience both in the role of the doctor, as the clinician, and as a key player within the multidisciplinary team. It is this particular area that I intend to focus this account around, following a particular incident on call, which provoked a role of the PRHO that I had not considered or indeed been exposed to in the past.

It was Friday evening, the wards were asleep, all was calm in the surgical assessment unit and my PRHO and I were doing one final round of the wards, before tempting fate and grabbing some sleep. On arrival at our final ward, there was an obvious air of unrest. One of the post-operative patients, a large, elderly lady, was in tears and the night sister was storming around the nurses' desk in a fury. During the course of the evening the patient had become increasingly uncomfortable with shortness of breath which we had treated with oxygen and nebulised salbutamol, and, following a CXR, furosemide. As a result of this, the sister appropriately chose to move the patient nearer the nurses' station in order that she could be kept under close observation. A reasonable manoeuvre, one might agree. It transpired that prior to the operation, the patient had made a considerable fuss about where she was to be placed in the ward: single-sex ward and by the window only. 'She knew her rights as a patient ... the government regulations said that she, by right, could request a single sex ward ...' One should by now be creating an image of this patient. These demands had initially been met by the nursing staff, but now this lady was unwell and the sister had taken positive action. This simple move had however upset the patient greatly, who in return had upset the sister and had woken up the other patients on the ward. So, our role? To restore calm, to ensure that the patient was effectively managed and to maintain a good working relationship with the sister.

This incident provoked several issues. The patient was anxious and upset as a result of the move and, one must remember, as a consequence of her operation and resulting heart failure; prior to surgery she had never experienced prolonged shortness of breath and this alien sensation in addition to the stresses of the day were obviously taking their toll. When unwell one is often irrational and difficult; did the sister take this into account during her moment of fury? Although not outwardly angry with the patient, the nurse presented with an air of antagonism, which the patient would have detected and subconsciously acted upon. Perhaps the sister too was under the influence of personal stress; as another team member this should have been acknowledged. Most importantly, however, this patient had the potential to deteriorate and thus being upset and in tears only served to exacerbate her condition. Our fundamental aim was to improve the condition of the patient; this, holistically, was not being achieved. Furthermore, she was threatening to make a formal complaint against the sister's conduct the following day. It was thus important from the sister's point of view to defuse the situation to prevent the necessity for complaint and to carefully document the incident in the notes. And for the sake of the rest of the patients, it was vital to restore a calm environment in which to get some sleep.

The key to resolution was the effective use of communication skills and to provide an air of calm, control and authority: leadership. As the doctor liaising between the two parties, it was important to listen to both sides of the argument and to provide support and empathy to each without being seen to be taking sides or passing judgement, but, in the same breath, trying to provide sensible reason and compromise. The power of a simple stroke of the hand on the arm of an anxious patient should also not be forgotten. All in all, a great skill, particularly at 1 o'clock in the morning with sleep deprivation and a growing desire to want to run off to bed! Calm was achieved. On the ward round on Monday, the patient was back by the window, with a smile upon her face. No formal complaint had been made.

This particular incident sticks in my mind as it highlighted the need for the doctor not only to treat the patient medically but also to provide support psychologically to the patient and the other members of the team caring for that patient, who for a variety of reasons may themselves be under pressure to perform to the best of their ability. As a prospective doctor, one's desire to treat the patient and family in a holistic and multidisciplinary manner often overrides the importance of ensuring that the other team members are working effectively and are themselves receiving adequate support. I had anticipated the need for a team approach and the pivotal role of effective communication but never before within the context of the dynamics between a patient and another colleague. Previously, my thoughts had centred around my *own* relationship with the patient, the family and the rest of the interprofessional team. This was an invaluable learning experience not only within its context, but also to observe how the PRHO effectively managed the dilemma – particularly in view of the time. In the words of our lecturer, we are the *chain makers* within the team. How very true.

What are you going to do with this patient?

'But what are you going to do about that patient, doctor?' It was a very real question addressed to the registrar, from a senior nurse on a surgical ward. We had just completed the daily ward round with the surgical team. Now we were sitting in the sister's office, drinking coffee and planning the jobs for the day. We weren't particularly busy, as all surgery had been cancelled due to yet another bed crisis. There were half a dozen patients, all of whom had been around for a while. The round had been particularly social in nature, not something a surgeon could get excited about. The team mood was one of frustration this particular morning; there was a feeling of 'there's not a lot to be done so I don't feel particularly motivated to do anything really … at all'.

'That' patient was a middle-aged lady, who had been on the ward for several weeks. She had presented with abdominal pain co-existent with nausea and vomiting. She had had pancreatitis secondary to gallstones, and a complicated progression so that she'd had a pseudocyst and now had a T tube and a pancreatic drain. However, she was returning to health, at least physically she was – her tubes had stopped draining fluid and her blood results were back to normal. However, looking at her, and talking to her, revealed something quite different. She continued to complain of nausea and wouldn't eat for fear of vomiting – she said she still felt 'terrible'. She'd had two gastroscopies to eliminate any cause for her nausea, but nothing was found to be abnormal. The interesting thing about this lady was that, although she was young and normally active, she had never shown any signs of frustration with being in hospital, or with her illness, during the long two months that she'd been in hospital. She never seemed to want to try and push herself, to restore normal function – the nurses would 'bully her to go to the bathroom and have a shower, if we didn't then she'd allow us to do a bed bath'.

The somewhat strained conversation continued:

Nurse:	What are you going to do with this patient?
Registrar:	Erm … do?
Nurse:	Yes, do …
Registrar:	What do you mean, what do you want us to do?
Nurse:	I don't know, you're the doctor. What about the nausea? We aren't getting anywhere; we can't get her doing things until her nausea is sorted out. Every day you go round the plan stays the same … 'continue' … are we going to let her carry on and on … with random weekly blood tests?
Registrar:	We've written her up for some anti-emetic, and we're doing a gastroscopy.
Nurse:	[Groan] … but she's already having anti-emetics, and anyway, that's not solving the problem. Don't we need to try and sort out why she's had this nausea for so long? She has already had two gastroscopies and they were normal. There isn't any cause for the nausea, is there? She's getting better, isn't she? It's not normal for patients to stay around this long, is it? Maybe she needs a CT head or something.
House officer:	I think she's depressed or something, I would be for sure, and her behaviour is a bit odd, maybe we should get a psychiatric referral, see a psychologist or something. I saw a lady once who had been abused as a kid, and she threw up every time she put something i.e. food in her mouth. Maybe the problem is that she felt so much nausea at the beginning, she developed a fear of eating and now it's a reflex reaction – food equals feeling sick. I think she needs a psychologist.
Registrar:	You think a psychologist is going to take one look at her – on a surgical ward – with tubes coming out of her abdomen. He will dismiss her and say, 'It's no wonder she's feeling sick!' Look, we're doing the gastroscopy, we'll just continue as we are, I haven't got any answers … [begins to walk away].
Nurse:	[Continuing conversation into corridor.] Listen, I don't mean to bully you, I'd ask Mr T (consultant) if he was here but it's so frustrating to have someone who is getting better really, just sitting on the ward, with no meaningful input. We aren't doing anything for her, it's a surgical ward, we like to have patients in, get them sorted out and then discharge, it's just demoralising and such a waste. We'll still be having this conversation in October … mark my words!
Registrar:	Oh well, I'll be gone by then, won't be my problem anymore! Oh listen, I know – it's frustrating for us

> too, there's no beds so we can't do any surgery today,
> I know what frustrating means.
>
> Nurse: Yeah, but you don't have to put up with her!

I sat and listened like a fly on the wall and, since that point, have reflected on the conversation, learning several valuable lessons for future reference. People talk a lot about the doctor–nurse relationship, and how it can be a positive, with one professional complementing the other, or how it can be a complete nightmare. In this situation, the nurse clearly had concerns about her patient and wanted to raise them with the doctor. She wanted some action rather than a passive 'we'll see what happens' approach. She was obviously finding it difficult to be patient with this lady, who wasn't easy to look after. The registrar didn't listen ... not properly anyway, and refused to show any empathy with the nurse's situation or agree with what she said. I think that he didn't do anything because he didn't know what to do, but didn't acknowledge this.

As doctors, we need to address the 'difficult' patients, and see them as whole patients, communicating with them to find out what lies behind the symptoms they complain of – simply ignoring them won't make them go away. The nurse went away from that conversation more frustrated than before, not feeling supported by the other members of the healthcare team. Surely it is important in such a case to work together, making a management plan, and measuring outcomes which can be evaluated, in order to prevent disillusionment and facilitate team morale.

It's only a rice cake

It is dark and damp outside and only the street lights illuminate the wet roads. Inside all the lights of the hospital are dimmed and it's with heavy eyes that finally having completed the menial 11 o'clock ward round tasks the weary and bed-destined houseman prepares to leave the ward. A final check at the nurses' station reveals no more jobs, but does offer up a box of chocolates and a packet of marmite-flavoured rice cakes. Tempted, the houseman helps himself to a handful of chocolates and then starts to delve into the packet of rice cakes.

'Not so fast!' comes the angst cry of the staff nurse who appears out of nowhere. 'They are mine, so get your hands off them,' she continues.

Somewhat taken aback the tired and therefore easily irritable houseman removed his hand from the bag. He was just beginning to enjoy the top-dog role that he had assumed now that his senior surgical colleagues had long since disappeared to bed. This was a bit of an assault on that position and to save face he sarcastically replies, 'All right, all right, keep your hair on'.

Determined not to be undermined by this upstart doctor who had appeared on the wards only eight months earlier, the staff nurse turns to the doctor and glares with a knowing look that without saying a word shouts out ... Mess me around and don't hope to see much of your bed tonight.

'Grow up, you're not the only one who's had a crappy day,' she snarls at him as he turns to leave the ward.

Seeing the imminent loss of face and desperate to retain the macho role especially in front of his shadow, the houseman leaves the ward quipping sarcastically, 'Night night, have a very pleasant time; as ever it's been a pleasure'.

The NHS is about teamwork; it is about different specialties getting on helping each other out and in the end providing the best possible outcome for the patient. Everyone from the Chief Executive to the consultants, housemen, to the staff nurses to the ward cleaners are under stress.

This story was very much the exception to the rule. The vast majority of interactions between different specialties were both productive and civil. This case highlights how very quickly there can be a breakdown in communication. While the houseman on call didn't get unduly antagonised by the staff nurse for the rest of the night, the case could have been handled in a very different way.

So how could this situation have been altered and what did I learn that will make my time on the ward easy both for me and for the rest of the staff?

First, the houseman could have asked rather than just assumed that everything on the nurses' station was for general consumption. This highlighted his opinion that since his direct seniors had gone to bed he could puff his chest out and assume their mantle. Why should he ask? He should just be able to have! This may stem from him being downtrodden during the day and finally seeking the opportunity to flex his doctoral muscles. The tired nurse was not the person to take this out on.

The ensuing reaction from both parties was one on many levels. Both the houseman and the nurse were tired and snappy. Neither of them wanted to lose face. While she shouldn't have snapped at him in the way that she did, the ensuing battle for the last word was almost like watching teenage kids arguing with their parents. The ability to back down and resolve the situation is vital to ensure good working relationships. You are not going to be able to get on with everyone that you work with but you don't have to be their best friend; just ensure that you are civil and able to get your job done. A simple 'Sorry I didn't realise they were yours' would have been all that was needed to avert the situation.

While the treatment of a patient was not involved in this case, it would be easy to see how this could progress so that a patient was dealt with sub-optimally. The nurse may be annoyed and continue to call the doctor back to the ward for menial jobs, leaving him tired, grumpy and more liable to make mistakes. The nurse could also become annoyed, disgruntled and less likely to do her job to the best of her ability. Thus the patient, who should be the raison d'être of all our actions, would suffer.

The conclusion: Be nice, understanding and realise that you can back down. At the end of the day it's only a RICE CAKE!

How old are you exactly?

There were various memorable incidents that occurred during my shadowing period; however, there was one incident that for some reason was more significant than the rest. I think that this event really holds strong in my memory, partly because it was the very first thing that was said to me on the ward by one of my future work colleagues.

Once I met my PRHO I would be shadowing for the next couple of weeks, he led me to the ward where I would be spending the first three months of my medical career, in order to meet some of the staff that I will be working with in August. As I entered the ward, filled with obvious apprehension, but at the same time masses of enthusiasm, I realised the pressure was on to make a good first impression. The first person we happened to bump into was one of the senior nurses. As soon as my PRHO made the introductions and explained how I would be their new house officer in August, the nurse just smiled at me and said, 'How old are you exactly?'

The reason why I chose this particular incident over the others is because, from that moment onwards, I realised that, as a house officer, I am sure to find it difficult recognising when to act upon nurses' requests/commands regarding the health of a patient, especially if I am not 100% in agreement with what is being asked of me. This potential dilemma only really hit me when this nurse asked me how old I was. It wasn't as if he said it in a menacing way, but more the fact that the first thing he said to me seemed to indirectly imply that he thought I was far too young to start being responsible for patients' health. Maybe I am just being too sensitive and I should be happy that I have maintained my youthful looks so far (although that won't last long working in the NHS); who knows, he might ask the same first question to every new member of staff. Whether it was a loaded question or not, I am not entirely sure, but it definitely made me aware that I am only 23, and my experience in dealing with sick patients, especially in the acute setting, is minimal compared to that of most senior nurses. However, although some nurses have more experience in these settings, this does not mean that they are necessarily always right, and at the end of the day we as doctors are the ones that usually take responsibility for actions and mistakes made.

I suppose that this incident made me more aware of the fact that trying to work alongside nurses, and other healthcare professionals, all of whom have different abilities and experience in their different fields, can be tricky but is vital in order to optimise the patient's care. I know that in some situations, a nurse could be my only saving grace because they have offered valuable advice in desperate times. However, on the flip side, one must not forget that five years of training means that we are also very capable in the majority of circumstances, and just because a nurse is very senior and experienced does not mean she is necessarily right. In the first couple of months especially, I think recognising which nurses normally give sound advice and those who don't could be difficult, but I am sure, with time, one soon learns whose advice and experience you can rely on. Ideally, doctors and nurses should be working in harmony, striving to provide great healthcare for patients. However, without that underlying respect for different healthcare professionals and their respective responsibilities, capabilities and experience, whereby every individual will be different, effective communication between us all as professionals will be impossible.

This incident will hopefully change the way I practise as a doctor as a whole. That day the nurse had made up his mind before even giving me a chance. He saw this 23-year-old medical student, soon to be their new house officer, and thought of me as just the next incapable newly qualified doctor that we have to get up to scratch before he goes and leaves us in three months anyway. Unfortunately, he is probably close to the truth, but that does not mean he shouldn't try his best to welcome new members onto the team, no matter what their position and experience. This event will hopefully remind me not to be judgemental about work colleagues, and respect that everyone has different capabilities and experience, and it is when various people's abilities are combined that you get a proactive, communicating and effective workforce.

Time to reflect

My shadowing experience coincided with an outbreak of Norwalk virus; highly disruptive to the running and daily routines to which I was supposed to be getting accustomed, this, I thought, was rather unfortunate. Without a single admission or discharge throughout the whole period, the well-known phenomenon of medical patients 'bed blocking' was only too well demonstrated, especially on this Care of the Elderly ward. It appeared at first that I would learn little other than exactly how frustrating such an outbreak can be for staff and patients (desperate to go home or for a long-awaited and life-changing pacemaker insertion) and being reminded of Semmelweiss's[1] pivotal discovery by having it drummed into me with enforced ritualistic hand cleansing every time I entered or left the ward. This was admittedly perhaps a very valid exercise with potentially many positive outcomes (or rather lack of negative ones) in my future medical career but with house jobs and medical finals looming fast such a simple albeit vitally important concept did not seem to justify the amount of time it was consuming.

With time to spare however and a ward full of patients it gave me an opportunity to reflect on issues that as a busy doctor I might not have time for and to learn perhaps not how to make my first few daunting days as a house officer more manageable but what it is that really makes a good doctor and what makes teams work well.

The most valuable experience of my shadowing was without doubt the day spent shadowing a student nurse. I was able to help give a patient a bed bath, dress and feed him. It struck me quite profoundly how the interaction with a patient on this very human level, at the level of very basic human needs, fosters a very special relationship between nurse and patient. There is more time to talk and to develop trust, to get to know the patient's true hopes and fears, to appreciate their well-being both physical and mental and importantly how it changes. On a personal level it was the first time I had been in hospital dealing with stroke patients since my own grandfather had had his final and severe stroke. Having seen him become (in appearance) just like all the other stroke patients I had previously come across, a shadow of his former self with only glimpses of his fantastic sense of humour and personality (which you now had to spend time around him to catch), it made me realise how valuable the nurses' role is. It struck me more than ever how much a ward round is like a snapshot and I was able to see clearly the potential and valid reason for nurses' frustrations when decisions are made on inadequate grounds and without their input.

The nurse-shadowing day was also a valuable opportunity to appreciate the difficult situations that they have to deal with. One patient on the unit was very distressed and complaining incessantly. He was difficult and abusive and it was remarkable to witness the skill and patience of the nursing staff in dealing with him and in remaining calm and professional.

It has often been obvious from both my own observations and time spent on the wards and from conversations I have had with friends who are nurses that the professional doctor–nurse relationship is often fraught and certainly leaves a lot to be desired. As a self-confessed idealist this is something I am uncomfortable with as I am conscious of how much we have to offer as mutually supportive and respectful members of a team confident in our own roles and in those of others and aware of where our own skills are limited. As tomorrow's doctors we are obsessed with good communication skills. We are very astute and alert to poor communication skills especially in our seniors and similarly quick to admire evidence of a good doctor–patient relationship. This has been primarily directed at patients. This is a great thing but implicit in being a good communicator is undoubtedly the ability to work closely and communicate well with nursing colleagues and other health professionals, to learn how to use their expertise to give us vital information about our patients which we do not have the time or the opportunity to develop ourselves and which helps to create a more accurate view of the person who happens to be our patient. This experience has made me aware of the extreme importance of good professional working relationships both for our own benefit and more importantly for that of the patient. This is something that I hold in very high regard and will actively pursue as a PRHO and beyond.

Note

1. Semmelweiss made the observation that doctors going straight to deliver babies having just carried out post-mortems (and not having washed their hands) were responsible for an increased rate of puerperal sepsis.

What I went into medicine for

Unfortunately our ward was closed due to an outbreak of Norwalk virus during my two-week shadowing, so I'm not sure how accurate an impression I've gained about the job in terms of workload, but I wasn't complaining – it was a great opportunity to have a break from study and I really feel that I've got a focus for my work now. We spend so much of medical school life working for exams and forgetting that it's all part of a bigger picture. I have come to realise that it is not just about knowing every eponymous syndrome in the book but about being good at the basics, organised and willing to spend some time talking and explaining things to patients. The shadowing course has boosted my confidence and taught me a lot in terms of the way I want and don't want to practise medicine when I qualify and for these reasons it has been extremely helpful.

The case that I am going to refer to is one of the patients that I saw when I was on call with my PRHO. Mrs X, a 90-year-old lady, was a classic heart-sink patient (which, incidentally, was why I think my PRHO sent me to see her!). She had been sent in via her GP with a suspected chest infection, which had caused her to become acutely confused, immobile and doubly incontinent. Her daughter was with her and explained that she had been caring for her mother for some time now and felt unable to cope with this recent deterioration in her condition. The daughter was very angry and upset because Mrs X had only just returned from a lengthy hospital stay where there were some unresolved issues about the standard of care that she had received.

As soon as I introduced myself I knew that it was not going to be easy – I had this worrying feeling that I would be with this patient and her overly verbal daughter all night and it was already 7.30. Mrs X was unable to communicate with me and so the only means of getting a history was via the daughter. I became increasingly frustrated as she talked *at* me, never seeming to answer my direct questions, and I felt as if I was getting nowhere and had no real idea what was going on with Mrs X medically other than what was given to me in the GP's letter. I was dreading my PRHO coming to find me and expecting me to have fully clerked and examined her when all I had elicited was the drugs she was taking! My PRHO was one of those very efficient doctors that I would imagine would have handled the situation a lot better than I did, and I felt really annoyed that I was having such difficulty – he always made it look so easy!

The examination (when I finally got around to it) was even more frustrating as every time I moved Mrs X, her daughter would shout, 'You're hurting her, doctor'. Being watched over as I tried to carry on was quite stressful and I was fully aware that I wasn't getting all the information that I needed, but I didn't really know what to do about it. I did as much as I was able and went to report my inconclusive findings to my PRHO, who was probably annoyed that he hadn't done it himself in the first place, as he was obviously going to have to go and see her himself now.

I wanted to use this example because I am sure it is a situation familiar to everyone. Having given it some thought I hope that the next time I see someone similar I will be better prepared – maybe it would have been sensible to ask Mrs X's daughter to leave as I examined her mother? I could have asked one of the nurses to talk to her regarding any concerns she had while I was with the patient? I should probably have interrupted the daughter more and emphasised the questions that I needed her to answer rather than worrying that I would offend her by doing so. In this situation the needs of the patient should have been my priority but being unable to communicate with Mrs X made that easy to forget. I have realised through this experience and from other situations that I have encountered during shadowing that translating the optimal management of patients into reality is always going to be difficult. It is easy to feel that the responsibility is all yours when in fact there is always a team of people at hand.

Somehow I felt that it was wrong that I was annoyed by this situation because I was meant to be acting as the caring, empathic doctor – it is easy to forget that doctors aren't superhuman and naturally find people annoying just like everybody else. The important thing is not to let it interfere with the management of your patients.

Aside from the above case one of the most important things that I learned from this shadowing was what sort of doctor I don't want to be. It is easy to forget how important communicating with patients actually is – even if it is just for a few moments – and I really noticed that a lot of the time patients' concerns and queries are overlooked. To use a very brief example, I saw a young man come in as an emergency with severe ulcerative colitis. A week later the surgeons went to review him with a view to performing his colectomy, only to find that he had no idea that surgery was even an option and certainly no idea what a colectomy involved. Our team had been reviewing him daily for a week and not at any point had anyone sat down with him and made sure that he understood what was going on. It is often a struggle for patients to get their questions answered on busy consultant ward rounds, which makes it even more important that their questions are addressed by junior staff who spend more time on the wards. When you are seeing sick patients every day I imagine that it is easy to see them simply as a list of jobs to get through but as long as I make myself think that any one of them could be a friend or relative of mine I hope to not lose track of what I went into medicine for.

Working within the system

Introduction

Students are the doctors of tomorrow entering a system already in place. They bring with them their personal ideals which have been developed in medical school and sometimes must learn the importance of maintaining their principles and values when faced with the exigencies and eccentricities of the healthcare system.

While the healthcare system continues to change and develop to reflect the needs of the community it serves, the students clearly identify areas of practice which, at best, continue to reflect old patterns and old styles of thinking and working. They recognise that as the most junior members of the team they will often have little influence on the systems that are in place even though they are aware of the need for change.

As the doctors of tomorrow students also have the potential to be the change makers of tomorrow. They are well placed to help us to see how 'the system' hinders the good care that they strive to deliver. They are adept at noticing without judging and their sense of purpose and enthusiasm is undiminished by the difficult practical realities they sometimes meet. Instead, they offer a fresh and positive approach to the situations they encounter.

Students are often surprised by the senselessness of some aspects of the system and need to remind themselves of their initial reasons for becoming doctors. They often correctly identify where the system needs to change and are sometimes overwhelmed by the expectations and demands that are placed upon them. Instead of becoming submerged by these experiences, they discover inner depths and find ways to deal with the system which do not compromise their values. They are often able to distinguish themselves as individuals with the ability to do the best that they can for their patients, their colleagues and themselves despite working within a system.

Their stories from the wards act as a reminder of the areas which still need refining and are often an inspiration to those who have at best become cynical and at worst forgotten the reason that they entered the vocation of medicine in the first place.

Up and out of the cocoon

My first venture into the radiology department – solo; a bit nervous, but sure I knew what I was doing. I approached a member of staff with my chin up. Perhaps my quiet tone belied my nerves. He looked me up and down before he spoke. I knew I was done for. A student? Requesting a CT scan? Well, I'd be a braver man than him if I dared to speak to a consultant. 'They'll tear you apart,' he spat, leaning forward with a rather menacing sneer. So I scampered away, feeling very foolish and about two feet tall. Stupid girl, stupid, stupid girl to have tried; certain that I knew the patient; I'd clerked her and knew her history best. Idiot!

Given time to recover a little of my dignity and composure, I got angry. What difference did it make if I am a student? He didn't give me a chance to fully explain my position, shadowing, learning to do the job. I was sent by my PRHO. The whole point is – yes, I am a student, but in a few months it will have to be me heading up that corridor to face a consultant and face the music. I'll look even more of a twit if I don't know how and get it wrong then.

I did go back, but with the protective shield of my PRHO to whisk me through. Perhaps it was inappropriate for a student to make a request, I'm still not sure quite why I seemed to cause such offence. There could be all sorts of reasons for the unfriendly exchange. I didn't explain my position clearly enough and, in my eagerness to appear unassuming and yet enthusiastic, probably gave the impression of being childish and inept. In the future, when my team is expectant of results, I shall have to be careful of how I ask for help so as not to close doors before I've even stepped inside. And of course take setbacks on the chin, and not be so precious and let my feathers be so ruffled.

On the Wednesday of our first week, I found myself on a ward where I hadn't yet spent much time. I was looking up blood results, watching events on the ward. The nurses passed the desk often, and would stop momentarily to talk to their colleagues. I overheard everyone who passed complain about the same patient in one way or another. I was curious as to how someone could cause such animosity on a ward, considering the patience that is normally extended to even the most frustrating situations. Later I discovered. My PRHO asked me to check how a gentleman was feeling. He was due to go home either that day or the following, depending on how he felt, so we needed an update on his progress.

I introduced myself, and inquired as to his well-being. I think perhaps I said four or five other words during our conversation, yet I was by his bedside for 45 minutes. I stood speechless as he systematically criticised every part of his care. From the GPs at his local practice, NHS Direct, the on-call GP and accident and emergency – no staff member was safe here. He delivered all of his scathing comments with a bizarrely benign smile aimed at myself. It seemed he wished to bless me, as a student, with some of his wisdom. I became more and more uncomfortable as the desire to escape from his 'tutorial' grew.

The main thrust of his unhappiness lay with the nurses who were working on the ward. He described how they played games with him; it must be how they kept themselves 'amused', he felt, making him wait as they went round the ward giving out drugs. This man seemed to feel that he should not be seen in turn on the drug round. Rather he should be seen first, or whenever he desired, on any whim, regardless of the needs of the other patients on the ward or how busy the nurses were. He insulted the staff's intelligence, and their motives for working in hospital. Inbetween the various character assassinations, he would occasionally throw in a condescending comment as to my being (a) female, (b) young and (c) a student. I'm not a particularly forward or aggressive person; however, on this occasion, I had difficulty holding my tongue.

This is an entirely new experience for me. I've never really disliked a patient before. I've been made to feel uncomfortable; I've been shouted at and ignored. I don't expect to like everyone I meet on the wards, but I haven't felt such unopposed dislike before and it worried me. At the time I dealt with it as I deal with most things that worry me. Cup of tea; good friend whose ear I can bend and I ranted for a little while about the incredibly unreasonable man I had met that day. Once I'd had my fill of ranting, I sat back a bit and thought about the experience a little more rationally.

The intensity of my response was a shock to me, though it passed very quickly. This was an eye opener. I don't expect this to be a regular occurrence, exactly the opposite. But it has happened, and it may happen again. I have heard patients complain about services before and, although it saddens me, I'd like to think that I'm able to see it as a learning point. For whatever reason, if someone feels let down by the NHS, by listening I might learn how to prevent a similar incident in the future. On this occasion, though I stood and listened, I was fuming inside. I certainly didn't use the conversation as an opportunity to try and understand him. I stayed quiet, at first just incredulous, and then angry. The more he said, the more ammunition I gathered against him. By this point it seemed rather foolish to try and get to the bottom of his unhappiness. I was upset myself and in no state to choose my words as carefully as would be needed. I felt a fraud when I finally excused myself, as he thanked me for listening. I later learned several of my colleagues had experienced similar barrages. I can't help but feel this man was genuinely unpleasant, and even if the entire NHS were rearranged to his liking, he'd still be unhappy.

I'm confident to say that I relish the thought of having a recognised role within a team. It's a feeling that has been growing throughout the clinical years of my undergraduate training. Having shadowed, I feel impatient to start on my career. It's a true step up and out of the cocoon of being a student. Taking off my security blanket, the short white coat that both protects me and mocks my inexperience. The responsibility is a double-edged sword. It's the push I need to step up and be professional, and something that terrifies me. Once the coat is off and my sleeves rolled up, there'll be no going back.

The patient as an individual

We had been running around all morning doing all the post ward round jobs. It was going well. There were two of us shadowing the same house officer and we were getting good experience of venflons, bloods, writing in notes and a lot of the practical organisational role of the PRHO. We were bleeped to pre-clerk two patients who were to be admitted for breast surgery for breast cancer. They had both come in yesterday to be sent home, and again today there were no surgical beds. In fact, for this very reason, they were sitting in the day case waiting room.

The pre-clerking that the house officer carried out was much like any other. The patient described the operation to 'have her breast off'; she had been coughing a bit and had upped her cigarettes to 40 a day due to the worry. The patient, the house officer and the two of us cram into the day case changing cubicle and watch a lady with advanced breast cancer having a history taken in a hot tiny cubicle with confidentiality, privacy and dignity afforded by a blue curtain. The house officer deliberated over the merits of a chest x-ray and sent me off to track down the anaesthetist who would be doing the list.

Problem one: List was due to be this morning and has now been moved to this afternoon. Anaesthetic secretary had no idea who the anaesthetist should be, would be or where they might be. Theatres were not answering their phone and I was left in the predicament of reporting this back to my house officer. We settled on doing the x-ray to be on the safe side. Were we doing this for our own sake and convenience or that of the patient?

There are still no beds and so both ladies due for surgery are having their post-op physio taught to them in the waiting room. The registrar arrives to consent and mark the patient. We pass the consultant to whom an opportunity to introduce ourselves never really materialised. He mutters something about medical patients and surgical beds.

During my shadowing I did not encounter or recall any clinical error, bad practice or an event that remained in mind, so striking as to feel compelled to write this reflection on it. However, it turned out that no surgical bed became available and thus for the second day the two ladies were sent home. It was a Friday and so I can only imagine how they got through the weekend or what happened on Monday. The reason I chose this to reflect upon was that it was an issue of the bigger picture. This was due to be one of the most important, life-determining events these patients would face and thus to reflect the impact of this seemed appropriate. The realities of clinical care in the NHS at a patient level were demonstrated as well as the crucial role that a house officer played in liaison.

During the shadowing course I gained a lot of hands-on experience of practical procedures and learned the value of politeness, patience and a personal visit to talk to the person concerned if requesting urgent investigations, etc. In all the chaos involved in admitting the patient, whose responsibility was it to explain the bed situation? Valuable insight was gained into the respective roles of the PRHO versus the SHO and registrar in matters such as consent.

Organisation seemed the key to the success (or not) of the house officer. If their role is smooth running of the firm then this facilitated effectiveness. Key aspects seemed to be to organise tasks geographically throughout the hospital, prioritise tasks and, if flailing terribly, ask for help or explain to the SHO in order to identify the most pressing of issues.

The issue of communication was really the key to the event that I described. The patients turned to the doctor (house officer) who was their first point of contact to explain the situation regarding beds. In a sense, the house officer was in the dark. With so many routine tasks to carry out throughout the hospital, keeping track of the situation regarding beds on a certain ward was difficult. However, a sympathetic yet practical manner and approach proved successful and I was surprised at how well the two patients I described reacted.

I learned valuable lessons. I gained further insight into the impact of a serious diagnosis along with the frustration from problems encountered within a 'system'. I saw first hand how busy house officers can get and how, in the running from 'venflon tissued cubicle three' to 'hasn't passed any urine in curtain eight', it is easy to forget that each patient is an individual. Liaison in the team was vital in order to prioritise tasks as well as keep abreast of developments, e.g. the bed situation. When in doubt, nurses usually knew the score, had seen it hundreds of times before and were on hand to help if asked. I really saw for the first time the role and value of good nursing care and that multidisciplinary care worked in practice as well as in theory and on exam paper answer sheets. However chaotic, unfair, hard and challenging the role of the house officer was at times, so were the problems faced by other staff and patients.

From this experience I learned to consciously make an effort in the rush of clinical duties to stop and think about the patient as an individual. I also realise that when problems occur this is inevitable and the role of the house officer is crucial in terms of communication within the team and to the patient. Practically one may be able to write additional facts in the notes – 'daughter taking GCSEs' – in order to recognise individual patients instead of slipping into the habit of treating 'the patient in two'. Continued learning and professional development are key and along with this was the reassurance that no one expects you to know everything on day one.

Shadowing gave me real insight and confidence and made me approach final attachments and indeed exams with excitement and a newly found light at the end of the tunnel. It made me appreciate the role and responsibility of house officers and the impact of this professionally and personally. 'If I …?' turned into 'When I …?' Shadowing turned what was a dim and at times very distant aspiration into a very immediate reality.

It's not all doom and gloom

The PRHO shadowing week provided a shocking but valuable insight into the harsh reality facing newly qualified doctors in the NHS today. My future job is on a busy surgical firm specialising in the upper gastrointestinal tract. The major thing that struck me during my attachment to this firm was the countless problems faced during a busy day/night on call.

The morning was taken up frantically trying to complete the daily housekeeping of the firm, before the rest of the world woke up to be admitted and the nightly onslaught began. In the afternoon, the pre-admission clinic was packed with patients sitting side by side waiting for their names to be called, only to be punctured with a needle before being told that their operation (that they had been dreading for weeks, and had arranged their lives around) was to be cancelled for yet another week. At the time all elective surgery was cancelled to accommodate and make way for the hoards of medical patients currently wedged fast in the system, due to the latest outbreak of a 'super bug'. This time it was 'Norwalk'.

On this particular night spent on call the hospital was extremely busy. By 5.30 pm the A&E department was stacked up with a backlog of patients, many of whom had been waiting to see the surgical on-call team for up to 10 hours. The situation became so dire that the bed manager negotiated with another major hospital to take the next batch of surgical admissions, as the hospital was bursting at the seams.

This led to countless difficult GP calls to the SHO on call, who, upon finding out that no further admissions could be managed, were unhappy about the 'unacceptable situation' and the fact that their patient would have to be referred to another hospital miles away from their home, where their relatives would have difficulty getting transport.

The theatres were still busy at 9 pm. All hands on deck, as the SHO tried to juggle a laparoscopic appendicectomy with an emergency abdominal x-ray (suspicious of obstruction) and numerous telephone calls from bed managers, irate GPs, overworked A&E staff and nurses on the wards concerned about sick patients. To further complicate the situation, the SHO in question was also scrubbed at the time, meaning that he was reliant on others holding the telephone to his ear and not actually able to touch any of his non-sterile surroundings.

Unfortunately, this was also a day when many individuals currently on the wards, many of them post-operative, became very ill. The theme of the evening was 'low urine output', often combined with hypotension and tachycardia. The corridors still rang with the echoes of bleeps and running footsteps even as the morning light filtered into the dimly lit wards and the hospital staff rubbed their grainy eyes.

From the perspective of an onlooker in these familiar scenarios, it became evident that the doctor played a number of different characters: negotiator (bed managers, GPs, other hospitals), counsellor (patients, relatives, colleagues), communicator (passing information between healthcare professionals and patients) and 'scrounger' (begging for investigations at unsociable hours).

As a fifth year medical student, it takes some time getting used to the fact that you are at the stage in your training when you can actually be useful to somebody. It was certainly a learning experience, after intense negotiation between the bed manager and the surgical team having to tell a patient in pre-admission clinic that the laparoscopic cholecystectomy that she had been losing sleep over, and built herself up psychologically, and negotiated time off work, and rearranged her childcare for, was going to be postponed for an indefinite amount of time.

I also learned many useful clinical skills during the course of this night, due to the fact that many patients had developed low urine output. I evolved from having only catheterised one patient previously to earning the nickname 'Catheter Queen' among my colleagues in one night.

At these times teamwork is one of the most important aspects of the job. Prioritising and delegating were other key words. Offering to help a tired colleague complete their jobs was an important lesson learned during that night. There are things that you can do to help take the pressure off others and ease the collective burden. This was evident when I watched a doctor writing up a drug chart at 5 am that a colleague should have completed before they went home.

This will not be an unfamiliar story, nor is it a new problem. A passing glance at any newspaper will confirm a new crisis in the NHS, but in slightly more sensationalist terms, and still the emphasis is on the inefficiency of the system or the dirtiness of the hospitals, or the gross incompetence or negligence of the staff, not the dire bed shortage or lack of regular staff that is causing the problems.

But it's not all doom and gloom. One of the truly valuable aspects of the NHS is the goodwill of its staff. Medicine still remains a vocation. Once you distance yourself from the administration, ridiculous unreachable targets and the bureaucracy, it is as it always has been; just you and another individual. It is finding the time at 4 am to spend a few minutes comforting a disorientated elderly lady. It is the encouraging stories, e.g. of the team nurses who, upon noticing the continual pressure on beds, decided to turn a room on one of the wards into a lounge, where patients who weren't seriously unwell could be seen by the doctors. The team painted it from leftover paint one of them had and hand-washed the curtains themselves so as to not to incur any further cost.

It's the little things that make life easier. That cup of tea thrust into your hand by the observant nurse; that hurried word of praise that enables you to muster up the last remnants of energy that you didn't know you had; and that patient who makes you think again.

There are no easy solutions to this problem but this example showed that good patient care requires good communication, a multidisciplinary approach, organisation, and time for patients to come to terms with their disability. Patients come in a variety of forms, both mentally and physically, and people's responses to something as traumatic as losing a limb can vary markedly.

I hope that this experience will help me put into practice those learning points mentioned above so that I will be able to provide a good service for patients and to be an effective member of the hospital team.

What lurks beneath!

It was during my 'interprofessional learning day' with a student nurse that I suddenly realised I was seeing something I had never seen before. For the first time I was given an insight into the true extent of NHS hospital filth. We set off together, the nursing student and I, to make beds. Before this I had assumed that between one patient leaving and the next arriving, bedside items such as locker, curtains, chair and table were thoroughly cleaned. I was made to think again, and not just because I was shadowing a 'student' nurse! We wiped the bed over with a soapy towel and then remade it. No disinfectants were used. Bedside curtains and locker were left untouched. Apparently this is normal practice.

Once the sheets have been changed, the outgoing linen is often placed on the floor before being bagged up and sent to the laundry. The bacteria from the sheets can then be transported all around the ward and the hospital on the soles of people's shoes. My suspicions aroused, I decided to delve deeper … and into the commodes! Protocols stipulate that commodes should be cleaned after each use. From where I was standing they appeared fine, yet when I ventured to look underneath, I found all sorts of biological matter, of varying ages, caked on. I very quickly got up again!

Barrier nursing requires all staff to don a plastic apron and gloves before entering the patients' room. These garments provide limited protection, however, the patients often grabbing onto those who are mobilising them and thus infecting their uniforms. Visitors frequently do not follow the protocols, thus supplying fresh germs to the patient and then spreading them around the hospital. Visiting the same patient subsequently in my 'student doctor' role, I observed the consultants too declining to wear the plastic garb. Does MBChB come with lifetime immunity to bacteria, I wondered?

The same sphygmomanometers are often used on all patients, including those being barrier nursed. In *The Lancet* (2000; **355**: 44), it was found that out of 50 tourniquets surveyed from a range of hospital departments, half were blood spattered, and all grew a variety of skin flora. Twenty-five per cent grew staphylococcus aureus and two grew gram-negative bacilli. I shuddered to think what interesting tropical diseases were thriving on the tourniquet in my very own pocket, seeing as it had been to Samoa and back on my elective. I disposed of it in the sharps bin for good measure!

Patient cups and crockery are all washed in the same kitchen as those from barrier-nursed patients and visitors. If the general standard of washing up is anything like that in my student flat, it will not be sufficient to get rid of obvious remains and stains, let alone microscopic ones! From my usual spot by the biscuit trolley,

I observed both a doctor and a nurse on my ward give cups only a perfunctory rinse before replacing them in the cupboard.

On yesterday's ward round my senior colleagues thoroughly examined four recent surgical wounds, each time moving onto the next without using gloves, alcohol gel or hand washing. Ironically, later on this same day I overheard my consultant and his team discussing the anathema of how MRSA continued to be such a problem despite regular staff screening for nasal carriage.

I chose this issue of 'grubbiness' as it surprised me so. The practices I witnessed seemed suddenly to explain why I had seen so many patients admitted to hospital going down with secondary bacterial infections. I saw various people exempting themselves from universal protocols and realised what a mammoth task it would be to educate everyone sufficiently to change their practices. I realised what a huge task the infection control team have on their hands and why there is so much emphasis on decent hand washing.

The student nurse and I discussed our own roles within hospital cleanliness. We agreed that it was our responsibility to wash our hands properly between each patient, and also to encourage those around us to do the same. For the first time as a PRHO I will have students learning from me and to teach by example would be a good idea. To confront the consultants would be too daunting a task, but we felt that perhaps if I and the other junior team members were more obviously clean, they might feel compelled to do the same!

From these incidents I have learned to encourage the use of barrier procedures across the board and to ensure that juniors and nurses around me are aware of their duties to prevent cross-infection. I will be more vigilant and intolerant of dirty hospital equipment and listen better the next time I am told how to properly wash my hands! The end result: my awareness is increased, my travel-weary tourniquet has gone, and I had a most enjoyable day with my nursing colleague! Perhaps everyone should be told to look beneath the commode?

For doctors to review, please

During a medical take one Friday evening, I offered to clerk in a lady who had been waiting for some time in MAU, for it had been quite a busy evening. This lady was 90 years of age and presented with increasing falls, worsening angina and a subjective account of 'black' bowel motions on a background of longstanding duodenitis. I duly took her history and examined her. My impression was that this lady had had or was currently suffering a gastrointestinal bleed, which was possibly contributing to her worsening angina and had perhaps precipitated her falls. At the time I saw this lady she was stable. Her BP was not significantly low (although I did not have a record of what her blood pressure usually ran at). There was no evidence of malaena on PR.

I presented my history and examination findings to the SHO on call, who was, admittedly, extremely anxious to move the lady onto one of the wards, who asked me what my impression was and we agreed that the lady seemed stable. I wrote up a provisional plan, which the nurse also incorporated into her nursing notes. We wrote up the plan in consultation with the SHO, who was, however, quite pre-occupied.

I then presented the case again to the house officer, who was taking blood from the lady at the time. I asked the SHO's permission to leave to go home as it was quite late and I was tired. I informed the house officer also that I was leaving.

The next morning, on the post-take ward round, a crash call was put out and the SHO and house officer rushed off. Some time later they returned – the house officer turned to me and informed me that it was the lady I had clerked in last night who had arrested. I felt mortified – I couldn't understand it. She had been fine when I had seen her. The SHO also returned looking dissatisfied. When I inquired as to what had happened I got a very garbled story – 'it was just a complete ****-up'.

I was told that the patient had had no observations done overnight. The night SHO had not been informed that the patient had had two episodes of malaena during the night either. While the team continued the ward round, I could not concentrate – I felt too upset. One of the other patients I had clerked grabbed my hand as we left her bedside and asked if I was OK. Luckily she was feeling a lot better than the evening before. I was so touched by her gesture that I found it very difficult not to cry.

I subsequently overheard the house officer recounting the story to the night SHO: 'She [meaning me] presented half the story to me and half to the SHO'. This cut through me like a knife. I felt this was an unfair portrayal and felt quite implicated – I had presented my findings fully to both SHO and PRHO.

I felt so responsible. Did the others also hold me responsible? What should or could I have done differently? Would the lady's management have been different had a doctor seen her initially? Surely a senior should have reviewed the case? But I am to be a doctor in a few months time. The responsibility of reviewing patients will be mine. Will I be up to it?

I asked the house officer whether the consultant would discuss this lady's case, given that she had just passed away. I had hoped he would say yes, for I really felt I needed to talk things through, but unfortunately the answer was no. I left the ward round, with my heart racing, still finding it difficult not to cry. I got back to my car and burst into tears. When I arrived back at home, I talked things over with my housemates – also medics. However, on Monday morning, I still felt disturbed and so I decided to go up to the ward where this lady had died, hoping to speak to one of the nurses involved in looking after her.

Unfortunately no one could talk to me at this time. Thus, I went to look at the lady's medical notes to try to make more sense of things. I was horrified to find that my entry had been the last before she arrested. I hadn't signed it. Moreover, to my dismay, a critical incident form had been completed. I began to read through it. It quoted the plan I had written in the notes. It stated that the clerking had not been completed or signed by a doctor. It went on to say that this lady had indeed had two episodes of malaena overnight, that nobody was informed, and that no observations had been performed between 10 pm and 7 am – the arrest call was put out at 8 am. It also stated that her Hb on admission was 7.1. Concerning the arrest, the incident form stated that the team was unable to find the store of gelofusine on the ward and that the suction equipment was faulty.

Now feeling that I simply had to talk to somebody about this, I tried to catch up with the rest of the team, but, of course, they were too busy with the morning ward round and were quite resistant when I brought up the subject. I knew that I had to do something and so I went to speak to my consultant's secretary, to ask if I could make an appointment to speak to the consultant about the case.

I was bleeped when the consultant had returned from his ward round, but was told by the secretary that the consultant did not know the patient in question, that he was very busy and that seeing him would really be 'for my benefit only'. I had come too far to be put off at this stage so I went and found the medical notes and went to see the consultant.

Of course, I apologised for the inconvenience. The consultant was reassuring about the whole situation, which I felt so responsible for. I felt so much better on leaving the office. I wrote one last entry into the notes stating that I had clerked the lady in and had presented the case to two members of the on-call team.

This remains for me the most upsetting experience of my medical training. I am sure there will be many others. It has made me realise how a patient's care can be compromised, not necessarily as a result of one mistake, but the cumulative effect of a number of errors. I still find it difficult not to feel responsible for what happened. It was the first time that I had been so involved in a patient's care, with such a tragic outcome. I feel that what I have taken away from this experience is a feeling for how essential it is for members of a team to communicate, whether relating to patient care or in 'debriefing' after a serious incident has occurred. I know that I will actively try to promote this type of communication in my working life. In terms of practical issues, I have not failed to sign a clerking since that day and now always write 'for doctors to review, please'.

The right to dignity and respect

I spent my shadowing week in an NHS trust, a hospital with an unfair reputation among medical students as being daunting and intimidating. I, as a student, have been a great believer in this hospital since my first clinical attachment there almost four years ago. It is a hospital with a community of professionals trying to do the best for their patients in an institution with limited resources and funding. I think that at its best these limitations serve only to strengthen the team spirit in this hospital.

The first few days went past smoothly and I began to get to know my way around the hospital and the systems in place there. I was very conscious of the need to write a reflective piece at the end of the shadowing and I began to analyse events during each day to decide whether I could write on that incident. In the end there was no question what I would write about although the incident passed without me once thinking of it in the context of this reflective piece, but it is an event I know will stay with me.

On my third day we had a new patient on the ward so we duly went to meet him and take over his care from the on-call team. The patient was a 74-year-old man with Parkinson's disease, who had been admitted for recurrent falls after an operation to insert a dynamic hip screw in his fractured hip three weeks previously. He was usually unsteady on his feet but on this admission the frequency of falls had risen to about eight times a day. All this information we deemed from the man's set of notes along with the damning statement for any patient written on the post-take ward round, 'Patient aggressive to nursing staff'.

The PRHO and myself went along to the side room in which the gentleman had been placed and as I opened the door tears immediately welled up in my eyes. Behind the closed door of the side room at the end of the ward was a frail man, who looked older than his years, lying on a mattress, the bed having been removed in case he fell out of it. The chips and marks on the wall usually hidden by the hospital bed were exposed, making the room seem more like that in a developing country than in an eminent teaching hospital. Worst of all the man had been incontinent of urine, probably as he was unable to mobilise without the help of at least one other person. He was lying in his own urine, trying his hardest to reach his glasses which had been placed out of reach, and had stretched over so hard that he was lying half in and half out across the mattress. The sight was pathetic and soul destroying.

After the PRHO and I had helped make the patient more comfortable and assessed him medically we left the room. I was still feeling overwhelmed by the indignity and shame that the man had been forced to endure. The nurse in charge of his care was outside to hear our verdict on the patient who she described as 'difficult'. I expressed how sad it was to see him lying in the room as we had; the resounding reaction of the team of nurses and doctors around was that I was too soft and obviously hadn't been doing the job for very long. I explained to them all in a softly spoken voice, not wanting to be confrontational, that I hoped beyond hope that I would never reach a point in my professional life where the sight would not shock and sadden me. I then said, 'Let's hope none of our loved ones end up in that situation'. The next day on the ward round I took heart; the room had been tidied and the patient was sitting up in a chair and appeared brighter and more alert and happier.

The incident taught me that I do care. That sounds absurd, but in the past few months of senior medical and surgical firms it is too easy to enter the stereotypical final year medical role looking on the wards for an aortic stenosis or a hepatomegaly rather than a patient. I used to think that I was becoming that person too. While shadowing, with no pressure of exams, on a day-to-day basis, it was easier to talk to and get to know 'your' patients and really care. This encouraged me; although the actual event was sad I was pleased with my reaction to it, and it did touch me and I was concerned. I realised that in a busy ward, with a lack of nursing staff and with increasing everyday pressures, the PRHO has a direct responsibility for each of their patients' needs, and the right to dignity and respect is one of the most important of these. I am grateful to have had this experience and to be able to call upon it in the future when I am again saddened by the lack of autonomy and the stripping of dignity that can too easily happen to patients entering a busy ward environment and use the experience for the protection of my future patients in upholding their basic human rights.

'Feel free to cope'

I intend to write about fear. Not the kind of fear which woke you up at night as a child, but the kind which keeps you awake at night as an adult. It's a gnawing feeling, which eats at you every minute, sometimes even through unconsciousness. The words we use to describe the sense it gives us are grand: impending, looming, ominous. But I think that they miss the point; the description should be more about the subject, more about us, and how it makes us feel: small, insignificant, overawed. This feeling can be only the beginning, as loneliness, hopelessness and despair can all follow a little fear.

Hospitals are fabulous places to visualise such trepidations. For me, the representation has always been (I think) influenced by Kubrick – the long, homogenous corridor stretching away from you as fast as you can run, the blank walls echoing your frantic footsteps. To slow is to lose hope; to stop, to admit defeat.

It doesn't, however, take very much to slow the corridor itself. I'm sure every individual in every group of medical students expressed, shall we say, concerns about the depth (or lack thereof) of their relevant knowledge prior to becoming a doctor. I'm sure every year someone says, 'We only need 50% to pass, but we need 100% in the job'. This year, as I'm sure in every other year, the message was simple: you don't have to be 100% but the system does. You work as a team to maximise strengths and minimise weaknesses. For me at least, the end of the walk seemed a little bit more attainable.

The incident happened during a surgical 'take' while shadowing. The senior cover for our on call was also our firm registrar, and as such we were together after the morning ward round. On discovering that his house officer was on that night, he said, 'Feel free to cope'. I thought little of it as it was not entirely out of character.

Later in the day, I asked my house officer why she had thus far not consulted the on-call registrar for managing some of the sicker patients we saw, instead opting to find other sources of advice. It emerged that 'feel free to cope' was the tip of the iceberg: the general impression she had got from him in their months as colleagues was to not bother him with questions or uncertainties, in other words not to ask for help.

Further into the take, as the majority of staff had left, all surgical patients in the hospital were covered by the house officer and registrar. Both happened to be on the SAU at the same time. He appeared in front of us and pointed grandly in two directions: 'These are the two sickest patients in the hospital. They are now your responsibility'. He then said that one of the patients needed immediate treatment with vitamin K. The house officer said that she had never done that before, so he gave what we, and he, thought were clear instructions. Before leaving, he left neither of us in any doubt that he wanted the drug given now and for it to be given by the house officer. Out of fear of being shouted at (not for the first time that evening), the house officer stopped what she was doing and followed the instructions to the letter; giving a 10 mg syringe of vitamin K slowly, which she interpreted as over two minutes, into the cannula on the back of the patient's hand. It was only later bumping into a nurse in the store room that we were told that vitamin K is normally given by nurses after having been mixed with 5% dextrose, at a rate about a fifth of the one our patient received. Having become aware of the mistake and the potential consequences, the house officer was understandably distraught, believing the event to be entirely her fault. I would disagree.

Whenever I am placed in a similar situation with instructions on how to perform a task, but with no prior experience (my first cannula, for example), I would ask nothing more than to have some degree of cover. That may mean knowing someone is there to help if needs be, or it may mean, as often, someone standing over you as supervisor. This need only happen once, but the confidence boost is immeasurable. I suppose it is my way of guaranteeing 100%.

In the case above, and in much of medicine, the 'system' refers to an invisible safety net. It is that which must be complete, certainly at the level of PRHO. The net consists largely of experience, and of the confidence that inspires even by its mere presence. The house officer confided in me that she felt unable and afraid to ask for help due to the nature of the command and the personality involved; the safety net was removed from under her by someone whose job it is to bridge the experience gap between them by making himself available in times of uncertainty. I would never advocate over-reliance on others, which can be easily self-justified as caution; I am aware of my own weakness in this regard, tending to need a bigger push than most before gaining confidence in something. As a PRHO I would aim to overcome this without extending to the other extreme of never asking for help: I do not see how, without the option of asking for support, the system is supposed to even approach 100%.

The Shadowing course, and that day in particular, were invaluable to me because it showed me the value of the safety net – of asking for help – and of, if necessary, providing it (the house officer was happy to observe me doing my first arterial blood gas while there were other things for her to be doing). I would hope that I can do the same: use the experience of others to enhance my own, yet being available for others if need arises. I also learned that communication plays a huge role in the 100% we strive for, and that it only takes a phrase, a sneer, or a derogatory tone to undermine the confidence of those behind you in terms of experience. From where they are, that experience is at the end of an ever-expanding corridor.

Hang on to the small things

> 'We have a 20-year-old male who has fallen off a motorcycle while travelling at speed. His observations are stable but he has been acting strangely. He vomited twice in the ambulance and could not stand up on his own. He can't speak and appears to have quite marked weakness on his left-hand side ...'

The paramedic is not speaking to me – of course he isn't. I am only a PRHO (or actually the shadowing student who was unlucky enough to be holding the trauma bleep) standing in the corner. This is a trauma call so I am officially the bottom rung of the ladder in this room; there are a surgical registrar, an orthopaedics registrar, an A&E consultant, an ITU registrar and the on-call anaesthetist all present.

> '... we don't know if he has been drinking or is under the influence of anything else. In the ambulance he became quite aggressive and he's a strong lad so watch out ...'

They get to work in front of me. The A&E consultant goes to the head and starts examining the patient; the anaesthetist is busy putting a line in. The orthopaedics registrar is feeling what looks like a horrifically damaged clavicle and the surgeon is placing a hand on the abdomen. I'm not doing anything. Why did I leave my patient halfway through a clerking on the ward to come to this? There are three other patients I should be seeing on the ward and ...

> '... and go and take this form down to radiology; we are going to need a head and neck because we couldn't get a good view of the C-spine ...'

What? Is the registrar talking to me? I have a job. I am to take this piece of paper and walk it down to the radiology department, put it in the hands of someone else and then walk back up here again. I leave the hectic room for three minutes and eventually come back in. The surgical registrar is answering his bleep in the corner.

> '… and how unimpressed do you think I am to be getting that kind of referral at 10.45 at night? … This should have been done hours ago … I know you are a busy house officer but I couldn't give a ****! Don't try and blame your registrar …'

One of the other house officers is getting a mouthful. It's then that I start thinking about this bloody job. Why have I let myself in for this? A glorified porter, we walk around the wards with our stethoscopes around our necks in the vain attempt to retain some feeling of self-importance. I don't know why I have come down for this trauma call. I might as well have not been there.

> '… here, fill these in …'

Ooh, some blood forms to write on. I sit down and copy some information onto the forms. I find the blood bottles and stick them in the bag, and then, for the first time in the last 20 minutes, I use my initiative and decide I am going to deliver the urgent bloods to the pathology laboratory myself. I walk out of the room feeling about as low as I have felt for a long while, and then I spot someone crying on the seat outside the resuscitation room. Can I help?

> 'It's my son in there and no one has told me what's going on and, and … and …'

I sit down. Three minutes out of my day are spent talking through what is happening to her son and trying to reassure her that he is in the best hands. I can't tell her much but I do try. As I continue my walk down the corridor I hear a faint 'thank you' from behind me and I smile. This job is worth it. We may just be a small cog in a gigantic wheel next year, but we are an important cog. We are going to spend hours and hours doing many seemingly meaningless tasks that someone with only half our training could do equally well. But it is the small things that you can do for people that you have to hang on to and remember will be coming round the corner.

Shakespeare wrote 'come what, come may, time and the hour run through the hardest day' and I think to listen to these words is good advice. The tough days will be very tough, and my shadowing has given me a taste of that. But what it has also allowed me to do is have that luxury of stepping back slightly and reflecting on my future job. I would not have had that luxury without shadowing.

As I continue around the corner of the A&E department I notice all the patient information leaflets on the wall. There is advice on diabetes, epilepsy and fractures but no leaflet entitled 'How to approach your PRHO year'. This shadowing course has given me the opportunity and time to reflect on how to approach and deal with next year. Thank you for the opportunity.

Haunted by the unwritten rules

Five long years ago, upon being accepted to study medicine at this university, I could not quite imagine the day when I would graduate and set to work as a PRHO. Halfway through final year I still was quite unable to picture myself on the wards as a junior doctor, working away in the security of amassed knowledge; for as much as I can absorb Kumar and Clark, take a history and examine, I was nervous about TTOs, imaging requests, whispering ward rounds, and complex systems for getting things done which seem to be understood by all and explained by none. As a fairly keen medical student I was haunted by the unwritten rules.

My first day in the hospital as a PRHO shadow was a whirlwind. I realised later that my firm had been on take the previous day, and the one house officer had almost 60 patients on 10 different wards. My house officer had not been aware that I was arriving (in fact the job for which I had been hired was changed, therefore the house officer I had arranged to meet was assigned to another student).

Because of first-morning introductions I missed the post-take ward round, and was thus not familiar with any of the patients. I was completely lost, running along behind a very busy firm who wordlessly dashed between wards. The house officer scrambled to keep up, and had no time for explanations. My offers to participate were politely but firmly declined in favour of speed. Questions were invariably met with 'you'll learn that when you get here'. I began to appreciate the feelings of bewilderment and loss of control that patients must feel during ward rounds; for they too have incomplete information, they too may feel dismissed or ignored when the overworked hospital staff don't have time to hear their questions.

When the ward round doctors rushed off to the next heavy file without so much as a word to the patient lying vulnerable in the bed, I would draw back the curtains and meet the eyes of the patient; a mutual understanding passed between us. I will never forget that feeling, and will work to try to reduce the helpless exclusion so many patients are faced with while we work our busy days.

At the end of a very long, bewildering first day I walked back to my accommodation feeling completely crushed and frustrated. I wondered whether they saw in me some incompetence that other hospital doctors had politely disregarded. My first day in 'real' hospital work had dashed my rosy dream of supportive patient contact, holistic medicine and teamwork. That day was the most discouraging experience I ever had in my medical training.

The next day I was scheduled to shadow a nurse. As always, the highlighting of multidisciplinary professions was valuable, not only for facilitation of communication and teamwork, but to understand the inner workings of the wards on which I will be a PRHO. I met several very helpful and energetic nurses, and I look forward to working with them. When I rejoined my firm the next day my house officer was much less busy, and began answering questions and volunteering information. Over the next few days he became more and more involved with training me to take over his job in August. He became encouraging and enthusiastic; I think he realised that I felt discouraged, and he truly made a heroic effort to teach me as much as he could. By the end of the next week he was sending me to answer his calls to the ward, make plans and write notes independently. I led the discussion with a lady about her dying father, and, watching him speak with families of other very sick patients, I was awed by his ability to find the right words, to simultaneously comfort and inform. Despite the manic pace of working on so many wards, he never failed to give his undivided attention, always finding a quiet place to talk and allowing the families to set the pace of the discussion. His professionalism and sincerity were inspiring.

I am looking forward to working at this hospital, and I feel much better prepared since completing my PRHO shadowing week. I saw how the frantic pace of busy ward work can interfere with patient-centred care, and I will strive to minimise this in my day-to-day work. I was also inspired by the kindness and dedication of the doctors and nurses I met there. I am honoured soon to be counted among them.

Stay true to who you are now

'Always remember to stay true to who you are now' – the words of the intrepid ageing healthcare assistant rung round my head on the wander home having earned my brownie points with ward staff on a day re-enacting holiday memories of bed washing, rolling old ladies' hair and tea rounds. Indeed, I could still say that medical school hadn't as yet succeeded in battering me into the classical egotistical doctor mould.

But what exactly is it that I should stay true to? Would the bumbling incompetence of student life not be best left in the pockets of my short white coat? Will I not emerge from graduation in the new garment of professionalism and knowledge?

First night on call, and any preconceptions of preparation are swiftly quashed. The venflon list is swelling exponentially and my competence to perform them is dropping just as quickly in the opposite direction! My 'befriending the nursing staff' tactic of a quick tour of the wards to round up any jobs before the rush only serves to remind them of the house officer's existence. A few inappropriate requests for other teams' TTA forms to be filled out are politely but exasperatingly refused. First lesson – just because a nurse asks you to do something does not mean that you must without question! I wonder if I might have naïvely been coerced into doing these 'urgent' tasks in my eagerness to please and follow the 'do not get on the wrong side of the nurses' wisdom!

Escape further discussion by a call to scurry down to the corridor to another ward: '72-year-old female, sudden onset shortness of breath, known COPD'. Flinging back the curtain we pounce upon our target. 'What do we do?' the house officer quizzes me. I stand gripped in panic, like a rabbit in the road, until from autopilot the ATLS protocol spouts out on cue and amazingly I find myself with an initial management plan before knowingly engaging my brain.

Sieving through the chronicle of notes filled with vague action plans and uncertain diagnoses to find the answer to what to do next is more complex. 'If worsens consider amiodarone.' Hmm … How does a lowly junior decide how best to tackle an unknown patient in the middle of the night? This time I was not on my own but how do you respond when everyone is looking at you for the answer, not just any answer, but the correct one and pronto? Reflecting on that incident now I know that this will be one of the scariest aspects of August. That dreadful feeling at the base of your stomach, heart racing and mind racking for a clue. The difference is that now I have thought about how I will respond when it's just me. There isn't always going to be a comforting doctor at my side to prompt and reassure in the quiet of the night. I see images of myself wandering round the hospital like a child with a teddy clutching desperately to my *Oxford Clinical Handbook!*

The day initially seems less daunting. Staff become more familiar and support more transparent. But dawn brings new challenges. Juggling priorities and requests. Breaking bad news and explaining the conclusions of the ward round later in the day to the baffled granny. It transpires that the key to success is, as I've often suspected, communication and organisation.

Our carefully constructed list of jobs is ambushed by an agitated son. 'Can you tell me what is going on?' The doctor's heart sinks. Mrs X has just been taken over and she makes a mental note to avoid outlying wards at visiting times. This saddens me as I can see his desperation to have a little more time to understand the complexities of the case, but unfortunately for him this conflicts with the doctors' desperation to complete her endless pieces of paper.

My previous eight weeks of student life had been spent at the same hospital and thus I felt I had less to gain from shadowing than most others. I could fill out the TTAs, navigate the computer system, sweet talk the right people in radiology and locate the nearest coffee vendor from every location. Pretty well practically equipped for working life perhaps, but the transition from student to doctor is the greatest challenge. I've been able to recognise my own weaknesses and likely hurdles. Vitally I have thought about how I'm going to cope when they arise and recognised that there are people to help. I've given self-approval to not skip lunch and appreciated that not only is it feasible, but that you really are allowed to leave at five!

Shadowing gave one final glimpse of hospital from a semi-independent per-spective. A reminder of how you want to do things and how you don't, maybe futile aspirations that will be long since ditched when that first pay packet arrives, but perhaps not. Perhaps these are the things you need to cling onto to remind you of why you wanted to be a doctor in the first place. Being true to yourself.

Day one, hour one, frightening experience one

Perhaps being greeted with 'This is the hardest surgical job in the hospital' made the first day a little more stressful than it really needed to be. Already with every new corridor, ward, form, job, new face there was the thought that (should I pass the dreaded exams) 'this is where I'll be, this is what I'll be doing, this is who I'll be working with, I'll be caring for these patients', thoughts that were generally accompanied by a mixture of excitement and nausea. Anyway, it certainly upped the already heady heights of trepidation, and maybe that is why the events of that first afternoon, which looking back on it now was not really so awful, at the time brought on a fresh wave of nerves and concerns.

On that first day the surgical firm I was going to be working for seemed to consist of three high-flying consultants (i.e. never on the ward), one registrar (also never available), no SHO and two house officers. This was a bit of a blow. I always knew it would be hard, but found reassurance in the thought that I would never be on my own; there would always be senior support. Now that comfort-ing support had been whipped away, and it appeared that the house officers were running the ward themselves.

This point was really driven home when it was noted that one of the more frail ladies post-hernia repair was a lot drowsier than she had been earlier that morn-ing, that her sats were dropping, and she was hugely oedematous. The curtains were drawn around her in that ominous 'something serious is happening here and these curtains will protect the rest of the ward from whatever is happening within' way that drawn curtains sometimes seem to have, and the house officers went over to see her. They sat her up, listened to her chest, checked her observations, struggled to take an ABG from her swollen wrists, pondered the drug chart, turned up the oxygen, looked at the ECG, ordered a chest x-ray and then racked their brains about what might be going on as a crowd of people gathered around the bed. And they didn't know what was going on, and they didn't know what to do about it (and they were two thirds of the way through their pre-registration year; how would I cope on day one?) and there didn't seem to be anyone to call for help; and that was the frightening thing. Everyone says that the day-to-day job of the PRHO is about filling in blood forms, sticking in venflons and running around chasing up the facts of hospital life. But now it seemed that maybe there was a little bit more to it than that, that people do unexpectedly deteriorate and that there won't necessarily be anyone around to hold our hand.

But, looking back on it now, with the benefit of two further weeks on the ward, and perhaps more particularly the benefit of seeing that same old lady sitting out in her chair the next morning having a cup of tea, it was not really so awful. The house officers didn't know what was going on or why it was happening, but they dealt with the situation calmly, and did all the right things. And although there was no one available from their team, they were able to ask for a review of the patient by the medical on-call team and when they came they had all the information they needed about the patient. The experience highlighted the fact that as a junior you may not fully understand why patients are unwell but that does not mean that you can't help them, and that basic principles should be applied. And that panic helps no one and is generally pretty pointless!

Over the fortnight it became apparent that the team was not as skeletal as it had seemed on the first day. There are three consultants, and at least one of them does a ward round every day; there are two registrars, and an SHO, and the heaven-sent nurse practitioner, who is the fount of all knowledge and I'm sure will be a life saver during those first weeks. And then there are the nurses, and the physios and the OTs, and the ward clerks, who all seem quite approachable and understanding. Which I suppose brought me back to my first idea that it may be frightening and overwhelming at times, but you are never on your own. And that remains a very comforting thought.

Shadowing has also reminded me, because it is easy to forget with exams looming and a limitless amount of knowledge that somehow needs to be stored away between now and then, that all this work is not just to get us through exams (even if it feels like that most of the time); it is to prepare us for the job we have chosen.

A good lesson

Lying alone in a dark stuffy side room – abandoned by the powers that be, by the busy nursing staff desperate to avoid the foul-smelling wound, by the busy catering staff who can sail by without a minute's thought and by the busy doctors who think they understand what is best. Can they even comprehend being in these shoes and surviving one day only to roll into the next with more needles, more tests, more surgery, more pitying disdained faces and more suffering? I mean – how long does it take to smile, to ask me how I feel, to spare a minute to explain or even give me a choice? I wish I was some place else – anywhere but here, anywhere but this dark stuffy side-room, anywhere but all alone.

Could one imagine that in today's NHS a hospital inpatient with a full package of round-the-clock care could really feel this way? Maybe yes, or maybe no; either way a good F1 doctor will spot these patients and give them enough so they are no longer that helpless depersonalised individual on a hospital ward. Perhaps this means staying five minutes longer after work and meeting your friends down the pub a bit late; perhaps it even means putting on a sympathetic face when all you want to do is scream and get out of the building and be a normal 'Joe Bloggs' again because you're fed up with moaning patients. Perhaps it means remembering why you wanted to be a doctor in the first place and actually doing that job justice.

That is the most valuable lesson I learned during my shadowing placement, and maybe the most valuable lesson I have learned during my degree, and what's more it reminded me why 10 years ago I decided I'd make a good doctor. And all of that from spending five minutes with a middle-aged man with a chronic disorder, who has spent so much time in hospital during his life he knows more about how the place runs than me. He had Felty's syndrome and was about to embark on his third debridement of the same perianal wound, and about his zillionth blood transfusion, and still had some medical student saunter into his room barely saying hello before they tried sticking large-bore cannulas into him. It took her a while to realise why she wasn't succeeding; the patient was tense, didn't want that cannula and didn't want the next transfusion. He communicated those circumstances by reacting disproportionately to pain. That medical student learned a good lesson that day; that medical student was me.

I think it is easy to get bogged down with trying to learn masses of medical facts and to reel them off at the appropriate point on a ward round to impress your consultant, or to think medicine is all about passing exams. But in reality medicine is so much more than that, and I think it's possible to do that job unbelievably well or unbelievably badly.

Having met the consultant surgeon I will be working for during my first F1 rotation he was kind enough to take 10 minutes to sit down with me to discuss career plans. He advised me that from day one I needed to think about standing out from the crowd and making myself a sellable commodity so that I could get the good jobs I wanted in the future. On that basis I need to think about doing audits and presentations when the opportunities arise. I'm not disagreeing with him, he speaks perfect sense, but I hope that not only can I be a doctor who can impress her seniors, but also one that can impress her patients. I am increasingly beginning to realise that (to be blunt) patients may at times make us want to rip our hair out; but they are also the fuel that will keep us going. Praise doesn't come easily in the medical profession and I should imagine it's quite easy to plug away in your job feeling out of your depth and not necessarily appreciated. So why do we do it? Job security, debt to pay off and a reasonable income all help I'm sure, but it's the odd comments from patients that brighten up the day and fill you with warmth inside, that help us get out of bed each morning and know we're making a difference.

And so without doubt the role of the doctor comes down first and foremost, as it has done since 425 BC with the words of Hippocrates, to the patients and their needs.

> I will follow that system of regimen, which, according to my ability and judgement, I consider for the benefit of my patients.

Just as we were reminded in the days when medicine began, one hopes that through all its stresses, strains and responsibilities, this profession will continue to bring satisfaction and joy to all who commit to it. I, for one, hope I can do myself justice.

> While I continue to keep this oath unviolated, may it be granted to me to enjoy life and the practice of the art respected by all men. (Hippocratic Oath, 425 BC)

Complicated

I have come to my reflections with some chocolate and a glass of wine, hoping that these will tease out the conflicting views about my shadowing weeks. I have spent time trying to make these thoughts solid, to hold onto some fleeting emotions. Ultimately I have realised that to try and give a taste of my shadowing is nearly impossible when faced with such brevity. It is all too complicated.

When I arrived on my ward the SHO said to me, 'The first thing you have to understand about our patients is that they are very complicated'. I didn't think much of it then, trying to look attentive and smile. But that phrase seemed to be repeated – 'Because of the complicated nature of this case', 'Obviously we need to think carefully, it's complex', 'She's complicated'.

And it was complicated, this job. A barrage of conditions I had never heard of, drugs I couldn't pronounce, signs I would not think to elicit. Simply doing the job meant thinking about practical things I had not considered – who do I need to ask to get this done? When do we have to know about these results so they can be discussed? How do I organise that test when I'm not sure even how to spell it? It was interesting to learn all about this rare medical problem that we don't often see, and good to time-manage, to prioritise. Then, at the end of the first week, my consultant said to me, 'You see, the medicine is interesting, but it is the social side that really hooks you.' Of course, this is what they meant by complicated. The people here had so much else going on, so many other things to think about.

The woman was in her late twenties, was missing a considerable section of her brain following surgery, was homeless and had no obvious friends or family. The team was unsure how long she had been in the country or what she had been doing before she was admitted to hospital. They knew she had sought asylum here and failed. Now here she was, in hospital, unable to use one arm and leg, and only able to speak in French.

French!

I realised that 'complicated' could mean 'quite scary'. I cannot speak any French and felt impotent at my inability to communicate with this woman. It seemed like such a straightforward thing, to ask someone how they are, or even just say hello. I was quite in awe of my competent and kind SHO, who conversed with this woman slowly and methodically every day. After several days I summoned up the courage to utter, 'Bonjour, ça va?', knowing full well that I couldn't understand any reply and this would be even more frustrating. I think somewhere I felt irritated. Six years of medical school and the absence of language skills meant I still wasn't good enough to do this. In response to my lack of ability, and others, the woman was angry and distressed.

I realised that complicated could mean difficult, could be used as a way to make difficult sound less derogatory. It was a way to distance oneself from the irritation of a situation, and prevent directing that irritation towards a patient. It was often said with a pause beforehand – this case is … complicated, as if another description was thought of and then discarded in favour of a more neutral turn of phrase. It's fine, I thought, I'm not expected to be able to do this, it's complicated. I watched my SHO continuing to talk and be kind. I saw that my consultant would learn two new French words before each ward round.

I think they recognised complicated for what it really was.

Complicated is not really another word for irritating, or scary, or practically challenging. On this ward, complicated generally meant vulnerable. It would have been so easy for the woman to be forgotten – she was unable to communicate well, destitute, disabled and emotionally stretched. Yet here a group of people worked really hard to make sure that things went well for her. And, more than this, they were kind.

I realised that 'complicated' people and 'complicated' situations are the reasons I have always wanted to become a doctor; this is the interesting bit! I get to do this (hopefully) in only a few months. I recognised when I was shadowing that I won't always be good at these complicated things, it doesn't look easy and I'm pretty sure I will make mistakes. Ultimately my team succeeded by trying to take the patient to be its centre, and by seeming to enjoy doing right by someone.

The word 'complicate' is derived from the Latin 'plicare', meaning to fold, to intertwine. All people are complicated; they hold a richness, present interesting and challenging situations. Complicated can mean difficult, it can be derogatory, but it can also be a realisation that we can never hope to contain the whole of another person's life; we can only hope to get onto their side and do our best for them. Personally, it's now the complicated bits I'm looking forward to.

Death

Introduction

One of the important responsibilities that health professionals take on is caring for people at the end of life. End-of-life care is perhaps brought into sharp focus by the transition between being a student and a doctor – not having responsibility and then being given it – and this often happens during the shadowing course, because for many students this is the first time they come into contact with dying patients.

Students describe their medical education as something of a lottery or a gamble. If something is going on and they are on the ward, they will see it; if they are in theatre or clinic, they won't. Students can also both avoid and be shepherded away from people who are very sick and dying. The assumption, from both staff and students, is that patients should not be burdened, or would not want to be burdened, by having students around. Experience of death and dying during their medical education is thus minimal for most students.

Students are often apprehensive about their involvement with very ill people and how they will cope with death; others have avoided even thinking about these situations. The following accounts all deal in some way with caring for a dying patient or dealing with death. For many students these experiences lead them to re-evaluate their role, to look again at 'medicine as cure' and to consider 'medicine as care', to examine the mystery of death and its emotional impact on those involved, including themselves. What shines through is their humanity; their wish to be the best doctor they can be for the benefit of their patients and their insight that for this to occur they need to care both for patients, and for themselves.

Life can change in a second

Life can change in a second; meeting the man of your dreams, meeting another car head on, meeting your breaker of bad news on the morning ward round. We can never know what lies just around the corner. As a medical student, I have frequently seen doctors telling patients bad news, and I have always felt privileged to be present, yet almost voyeuristic; nothing more than a silent, sympathetic, staring witness. I have always felt sad for the patients, but detached. During my shadowing week, I found myself unexpectedly affected by seeing a patient being told she had inoperable bowel cancer.

She was sitting up in bed. Her cheeks were hollow, her hair limp and tired. There was no sparkle in her eyes, no flesh on her desperately thin frame. She smiled at us, looking for signs of hope, for good news, for any clues from our body language as to what was coming next. I drew the curtains round as we lined up as if for battle; doctors versus relatives, patient in the middle, nurse hovering between factions to ensure fair play. Her father stood next to her, but he was too old now to keep his daughter out of harm's way. Her husband was her guardian angel, standing at the foot of the bed; out of eye contact with everyone except his beautiful wife.

'We have failed this patient' was my only thought. She had presented over 15 months ago with bowel symptoms, and was fully investigated. How had her cancer not been found? Somehow, I felt as though I was personally responsible. She was only 51; my mother's age.

All eyes were on the consultant. What would he say? He was gentle, clear, genuine and faultless in his delivery. Brilliant, in fact, given the circumstances. He had not removed the tumour, he said; it would have been too big an operation for her in her current frail state. He said that the cancer was not just in the bowel; the tumour had stuck her bowel to her uterus, and had spread to her liver and both sides of her diaphragm. He wished he could have been standing there telling her that he'd removed all the cancer, he said, but all he had done was to bypass it. He had not removed anything at all.

I didn't know where to look. I realised my heart was pounding and my eyes were welling up. She never moved her gaze from the bearer of bad news; her angel of death. Her life had changed in a second. Was she still listening to him? How could she take all this in? 'Advanced cancer' … 'extensive disease' … 'some chemotherapy might help' … 'the oncologist will come and see you' … '*I wish I was standing here telling you that I have removed all the cancer*' …

I looked around the characters in this scene, putting myself into each person's shoes in turn. How was the patient so gentle and accepting? Why wasn't she angry? Her husband stared at the floor. I looked at her father who was looking at me. I saw no anger, no disbelief, no blame, just deep sadness and grave understanding in his eyes. Should I look down, look away, smile one of those hopeless half-smiles of pity? Was he looking for a glimmer of hope in my eyes, trying to shake himself out of this bad dream? I held his gaze a moment longer, and then he looked back to his daughter. Is it true that the eye is the window to the soul? Could he see my genuine sadness, coming from that part of the heart so deep that it must actually be in the stomach, because it was making me feel sick. His daughter was the same age as my mother. I tried not to let my imagination rewrite the scene with a different character playing the lead.

I was clutching the patient's notes, but scribbling; 'Obs stable, apyrexial, patient not in pain, diagnosis explained, husband and father present' seemed rather a callous oversimplification of the situation. How could I write 're-site cannula, 'phone oncologist, refer to dietician' on the jobs list, while this lady was trying to imagine how long she had left in this world? I would write later.

We seemed to be in the cubicle forever – the medical trio and the family trio – staring at each other. Finally, the full, unabridged version of the bad news had been broken. The patient had nodded, smiled gently, said 'yes', throughout. She looked so thin, so vulnerable, so helpless. The consultant asked if she had any questions.

'Will I be able to go home again at all'? asked the patient. '*Will I die here in hospital?*' was what she was really asking. When she heard she should be well enough to go home, and could have chemotherapy as an outpatient, she beamed a smile so radiant that her eyes almost twinkled.

How had she readjusted so fast? She had been hoping to hear that all her tumour had been removed; she was told it had spread everywhere. But there was no anger, no blame, no recriminations, no tears; not yet, anyway. Just a dazzling smile across her pale, thin face when she heard that the end was not here and now; she would be able to go home. How had she reset her expectations of life so quickly?

We left the curtains closed to protect the shell-shocked trio. The father and husband powerless now to protect this woman whom they loved so deeply. What words of comfort would they find to offer each other now that their lives had been turned upside down in a few seconds? Were the magic curtains containing the conversation from the other three patients in the bay?

Were they thanking their lucky stars it wasn't them? Would they know what to say when the curtains were opened again?

Postscript

Her condition deteriorated and she was taken to ITU two days after I wrote this. I found myself going there every day to see how she was doing, until I realised that she was never going to go home again, and then I couldn't bear to go any more.

The 'learning need' to be developed in my PRHO year would be to maintain perfect poise on the knife-edge between emotional involvement and professional detachment. Fortunately, however, most of us are human beings, not machines, and falling either way is inevitable and acceptable. It is important, from an emotional survival point of view, to try and predict which patients affect us most, and not to fall too far … And also not to feel personally guilty for things which cannot be changed.

I can still hear her hopeful little voice: 'I was hoping you were going to say you'd taken it all out'. And I can still see her brave, dazzling smile at the thought of going home.

Too much grey

> Click.
> Black and white and grey.
> Click.
> Black and white and grey.
> Click.
> Black and white.
> And grey.
> Too much grey.

The CT cross-sections are flicking up in quick succession, scrolling through liver, kidney and into the colon. Or at least where the colon ought to be. But there's just amorphous greyness eating away at the familiar structures. Too much grey.

I'm sitting there, at the back of the MDT meeting, feeling queasy. Is it motion sickness from the whizzing by of the histology samples or is it because I know that this person is going to die? I've never even met them; they're just a name on the word-processed list in front of me but they're dying and I know it. And very likely *they* don't know it yet. I look up at the monochrome slices of this man, looking into his middle and into his future, and I feel so privileged and so ashamed. How can five years of lectures and exams give me the right to see this? Why do I have to see this? Why do I have to know?

Knowledge seems to me to be the hardest burden that a doctor carries and an F1 is no exception. We spend all our time afraid of what we don't know, what we've forgotten, what we've never learned. But they aren't the bits that get us. The bits you don't know can't follow you home and keep you awake at night. It's what you do know that does.

We knew Alice was going to die. Alice's husband knew she was going to die. Alice's mother knew she was going to die. And Alice knew she was going to die. And we all knew why. Alice had stopped eating. Years ago Alice had been diagnosed with tonsil and tongue cancer. She'd been treated and apparently cured but what remained was not cancer but perhaps something worse: the ghost of it, the haunting thought every morning when Alice woke that it was back. Hiding herself away in her house each day with that spectre was too much. Alice decided to beat it in the only way she knew how: she'd stop the cancer killing her by dying before it had a chance, dying through her own force of will, by not eating. That way she had the power.

A week ago, when I started my shadowing, she'd been sitting up and chatting as we tried to get a cannula in. Now she was unconscious and suddenly *we* had the power. She'd refused an NG tube and any kind of nutrition but now she was classed as incompetent and all the doctors had to do was to invoke common law and feed her 'in her best interests'. But they didn't. They spoke to Alice's family and decided, with them, not to be heroic. They would not drag her back to consciousness and competency with calories, only for her to refuse to live all over again. Sitting in the relatives' room with its pot of plastic pansies I watched as her mother decided to lose the only child she had. I watched as her husband said he would not visit her now till she was gone. And I watched as the consultant showed me how to talk to relatives by saying almost nothing at all. Through all this my F1, the 'me-to-be', just sat there and recorded it all in the notes, silently. It was recorded that we knew, we all knew, Alice would die very soon, and we were letting her.

A few days before this she had become confused and I watched my F1 making life harder for himself by trying to keep her thinning pubic hair covered with the sheet as he drew blood gases from her groin. It's so easy to forget that there's a woman attached to the end of the needle and that a falling Glasgow Coma Scale does not allow a fall in respect. But this unassuming, usually laid-back F1 did not forget, tangled, as he was, in bits of bed sheet and cotton wool. Please, please, please, I whispered inside, let that be me next year; sometimes making life harder for myself in order to make it easier for someone else.

My shadowing period ended the same day that they decided to let her die in that room with the plastic pansies. I left a card for the ward staff and I left Alice.

Because I didn't see her die, I'm rescued from knowing that it has happened. But it will have happened by now. On a ward, surrounded by people who could not eat because of the cancer they were dying from, Alice died because she would not eat because of the cancer she did not have. When other people die it is hard because often we do not know the way to save them, but with Alice it was so hard precisely because they *did* know how to save her. They knew and they knew that they couldn't do it.

There was no grey area on Alice's CT, but there was grey all around her. There was no black and white, no clear-cut blood test to be treated or bone to be fixed. It was the kind of case I would have relished four years ago in an ethics tutorial: all blurred boundaries and shades of grey. But in August it stops being an ethics case; it becomes a woman in front of me.

And I will take the blood gas that shows she is so sick.

And I will write the record that says we will not save her.

And I will work in this job where there is too much grey.

Learning to let go

An elderly lady with learning difficulties and epilepsy, admitted in status epilepticus, arrests during the night. She is 'brought back' to lie for two days in a coma, her oxygen saturations hovering around 80%, her brain probably already too starved of oxygen to appreciate the activity going on around her; the daily hustle and bustle of life on a hospital ward. She exists in limbo, waiting to fade away into the unknown. While she walks the line between life and death the term DNAR is bandied about and, while the lunch trolley arrives clattering on the ward, someone asks about the relatives. Into this already heart-wrenching scenario another note of despair is added – she doesn't have any. She has lived her life until now in a nursing home, with no awareness of the world that is happening beyond her four walls and the life that she, by a cruel twist of fate, has been denied.

The DNAR notice is signed, the term 'in the patient's best interests' is mentioned and the nursing home informed. The curtains are drawn around the bed and the PRHO with his shadow leaves to attend to those patients who still have a tenuous grasp on life.

The shadow, while trying hard to concentrate on the day's tasks, finds her thoughts constantly straying back to the curtained bed on the ward at the end of the corridor, where the patient that she had chatted and laughed with only a few days before is now fighting for her life. And, sure enough, the time the shadow is dreading arrives, and the PRHO is bleeped to the ward with the phrase ... 'We think she's slipping away'. We stand around the bed, watching the oxygen saturation monitor creep slowly downwards, the heart monitor change from its regular reassuring bleeps to a chaotic jumble of spikes and lines, and our patient fight for breath. All too quickly, although it seemed hours at the time, she moves from this life to whatever awaits her elsewhere, the transition noticed only by those of us privileged, or unlucky enough, to be present. On the crowded ward, with patients and relatives sitting feet away, talking happily, with no idea what is happening behind the curtains, our patient dies without the family and friends around her that we take for granted all too regularly. Her death is certified and documented, the words 'Rest in Peace' inscribed, and a line drawn beneath signifying the completion of the medical care of our patient and the ending of our brief role in her life.

Having been fortunate enough never to have witnessed the process of dying, I nevertheless naïvely assumed that when the time came I would manage – that I would know the right thing to do, would be strong enough to do my job and move on. Anatomy cadavers and patients to certify had never provoked any other response in me than an impersonal respect for the dead. However, the episode I have just described, the first time I sat by watching a person I had come to know dying, shattered my confidence, causing me to question whether I could act objectively in these situations. I have thought about what happened many times, trying to answer questions such as why did this event affect me so much when I have always believed myself capable of acceptance and rational thought and behaviour in a clinical setting. Why has all the combined training of the many doctors under whose care she died been unable to provide a solution for her to go on living, and why is her right to live or die decided by her doctors, when surely only she should be able to say, 'This is what I want'?

The minutes that I sat with her, holding her hand and waiting for her to die, feeling helpless at our inability to do anything else for her and guilt for the paternalism that we had inflicted upon her, the inevitability of death that had always seemed so far away confronted me with my guard down. Nothing in my training had prepared me for this – the reality of death and my own reaction to the process being played out before me. However, as I sat with her, feeling scared, angry and defeated, I realised that there *was* more I could do for her – I could be with her at the end.

I have since come to realise that although death is an inevitable part of the job and I hope never to become immune to it, I will eventually find a coping strategy while recognising my own vulnerability. I have accepted that I will never find it easy but I have attained a deeper understanding of my role in the care of my patients in both life and death. I know that I will remember my patient and the gift that she gave me – to understand, in the future, that being there at the end is providing the last final service that we can offer, not a giving up of responsibility. That day I felt that I would never be able to deal with death objectively, hardly the prerequisite of a good doctor, but I now feel that the vulnerability that we feel when faced with a dying patient may in fact make us better doctors than we realised we could be in making us drop ever so slightly the façade that we have built up around ourselves.

Consequently I feel that I finished the shadowing course with a deeper understanding of my role as a doctor, an understanding that theory could never have prepared me for. That, despite the multitudes of drugs and interventions available, there are times when it is kinder to the patient to let them go without suffering and with their dignity intact. That we cannot cure all our patients and that death is inevitable, but that in these situations being with them at the end benefits both them and ourselves.

Reflecting on this event and my role in it, again and again I come back to one issue – that, despite my feelings of inadequacy and inability to help her medically when her time came, I hope that she knew my gift to her; that at the end I held her hand and grieved for her, glad that her death was peaceful and that I was doing what little I could.

Whatever you feel most comfortable with

Early on in my PRHO shadowing period I developed a deep sense of admiration for the house officers I was following. Ahead of us mere students by just one year; the nights on take, weekends on ward cover and venflons, venflons and more venflons had rendered them truly competent and confident working professionals. Amazing! So this was how I had to be within a year. This was what I would be doing. This was how confident I would feel. All this would just be second nature ...?

We wandered around the ward, checking observations, sharing the odd joke with a patient and chatting politely to their families. We would then sit at the computer for a while and order x-rays and blood tests, prescribe fluids, rewrite a few drug charts. At first I was simply confused. Erm … what dose of furosemide do I write up? And is that bd? Oh, in the morning … of course! Where do I find those pink forms again? Electronic ordering – what a joy. No scribbling out blood forms. Life made simple. Actually … could you tell me your password again? Thanks.

But it was on my fourth day of shadowing, the Monday of the second week, that this routine was thrown into disarray. Within just a few hours three of our patients passed away. I do not think any of these deaths was unexpected; it is a Care of the Elderly ward and these ladies had all been there for some time, not really getting any better, just hanging on. Our consultant had long and careful discussions with daughters, son-in-laws and sons during the preceding Friday's ward round concerning what we should and should not be doing at this time. Appropriate care had been agreed, unnecessary treatments withdrawn. But, of course, no amount of expectation or preparation can take away the loss felt when a loved one dies. The ward was filled with distraught relatives. Two nurses walked past us, eyes filled, cheeks wet. They had been sitting with a patient and her family while she closed her eyes and slowly drifted away. She had been one of their favourite patients.

This was a Care of the Elderly ward. These nurses and doctors had all looked after patients who had died before now, and they would do again. But I could see they were affected by each of these deaths. Some more than others, depending on how involved they had been with that person's care. But, for each of them, dealing with these situations was not just part of the daily routine. Clearly there were certain aspects of the job that would simply never become easy to deal with, second nature, a breeze.

My PRHO and I had to go and see one of these patients to confirm her death. The curtains around her bed were drawn. 'Should I go in?' she whispered nervously to two nearby nurses. 'Is her son still with her? How is he?' 'I hate having to do this,' she confided. We slipped in through a gap in the curtains. The son looked up at us, tears in his eyes, and smiled. The PRHO introduced us both. 'Thank you,' he said. 'Thank you both for everything.' We smiled. We all stood for a few moments and looked down at her peaceful face. The son talked about his mother for a while. She had been ready to go. It was the right time for her. He cried some more and we listened. The PRHO touched his hand. He clung to hers. 'I'm afraid I have just a few official things to do,' she told him quietly. 'Should I leave?' he asked. 'Whatever you feel most comfortable with, it's up to you. It will only take a few minutes'. 'I'll stay …' he replied '… if that's OK?'

Of course it was OK. My PRHO may have been a bit nervous about disturbing this lady's son. She had told me she hated doing this. Who wouldn't? But by the bedside she seemed so confident. So poised. She did everything expertly, professionally, respectfully. She then turned to the son. 'Thank you,' she said. 'Are you all right? … Do you have any questions? … You can take as much time as you need here,' she reassured. He smiled. Gripped her hand once more. 'Thank you. Thank you again.'

I was overwhelmed. This man had been so grateful for her kind words. Perhaps she had felt uneasy, but it really did not show. I made a mental note; this was how I wanted to deal with this kind of situation in five months time. This was the kind of house officer I wanted to be. I could see that the job was still going to challenge me, even when I had learned how to log into the computer and order U&Es and LFTs with my eyes shut. Even once I could recite the route and dose of all the common diuretics in my sleep. Of course, there is more to it than all those things. I finished my PRHO shadowing week inspired and still filled with admiration for these fantastic doctors. I hope that, despite the inevitable times of stress, fatigue and frustration that I will face during the coming year, I will not forget that this is the kind of doctor I aspire to be. I hope that this time next year I will be able to look at myself and know that I am being that kind of doctor. I realise that, come August, I will still have an awful lot to learn.

Could I object?

'Are you the medical student?' I was asked as I sat one evening, writing up my examination findings on the medical admissions unit. I had just begun to wonder what I should do if the registrar to whom I had presented the lady's history did not reappear, having horrible images of her collapsing quietly in the corner of the room because I hadn't recognised her as being at risk of doing so.

'Yes' I beamed, slightly surprised at the unusual interest invested in my lowly presence.

'We need your help, come with me' was the response.

Very intrigued, I followed immediately, being careful to leave my clerking in a prominent location on the desk, in case anybody needed any information about the lady to whom it referred.

Walking rapidly out of the unit, my mind pondered the possibilities ahead, until its thoughts were interrupted. 'You get to do some chest compressions.'

OK. Calm. You can do this. Two finger widths above the xiphisternum, using heel of hand, rate 100 per minute, theme tune to the Archers. Barely breathing, I was aware of being detached from myself. The terror of pushing too hard, breaking ribs, or worse not pushing hard enough to circulate blood, the terror of letting this person die, was suppressed before it was allowed to surface. Calmly, we marched onto a ward and into a bay.

The curtains were pulled closed around every bed except the middle bed on the left-hand side. There, a man lay on the ground. An assortment of equipment surrounded him, and a man knelt at his head squeezing oxygen into his lungs via a bag and mask.

'We've got an output for the moment. Would you like to take over the breathing?' 'Sure,' I heard myself say. Don't panic. Just squeeze the bag at the appropriate times.

'A nurse found him slumped in his chair about two minutes after she'd given him his tablets. He is known to have lung fibrosis, and was preparing for discharge in the next couple of days. When found, he was in VF, so we shocked him into pulseless VT, then into sinus rhythm.'

As I pushed oxygen into the gentleman's lungs, it struck me that behind each of the five curtains in the room was a person. Each person could hear everything that was going on in the bay, and may be interpreting the things they heard to form an image of what was happening. Each person may also have got to know and formed a friendship with this man. Each person may also be feeling vulnerable themselves and more aware of their own ill health by virtue of being in hospital. I wondered what impact this incident would have upon them.

'We need to get some blood gases. Would you like to take some?' 'Sure.' I handed the bag to the anaesthetist who took over the breathing, and was handed a blood gas syringe. Feeling for a femoral pulse, I was oddly surprised by how cold the man felt. The pulse felt of good volume, and I obtained a sample of blood.

Now that things seemed to have stabilised, arrangements were made for his transfer to the intensive care unit. The anaesthetist ensured that he had all the equipment he would be likely to need in case of an unforeseen event occurring during transit, such as the lift breaking down.

Once in ICU, I was asked to take another blood gas. Again, I felt for the femoral pulse. I could not locate it. Putting it down to lack of experience, I continued to feel. He felt very cold. Eventually, I found a very weak pulsation in the groin. 'He has a very weak pulse,' I announced, looking at the cardiac monitor in time to see a rhythm change.

A man beside me immediately began chest compressions, and somebody was preparing the defibrillator when the anaesthetic registrar entered. 'I think we should stop. The cardiologist has found little evidence of any left ventricular function, and his pupils have been dilated and unresponsive for quite some time now,' she announced. 'Does anybody have any objections?'

A series of 'nos' echoed around the room. My head sat firmly still, my lips closed. Could I object? Not doing so would result inevitably in this man's death. But was he alive now anyway? He was unable to breathe for himself, with likely brain damage, and a poorly functioning heart. But how could I let this man die?

I did not know what he would have wanted, so could not consider his autonomy. Was letting him die better for him than putting him through further resuscitation? What benefits would resuscitation bring? All the evidence suggested it would lead to very little benefit. What harm would it cause? It is an unpleasant and undignified, somewhat traumatic process. In view of this, when the registrar's expectant gaze fell upon mine, I shook my head.

The gentleman's family had arrived and the situation had been explained. They entered the room as we left, and sat with him.

Upon my return to the medical admissions unit, the lady who I had clerked earlier sat happily awaiting a bed.

We, as members of a clinical team, are in an extremely privileged position. We have the opportunity to make a difference at every stage of a person's hospital experience. It is this opportunity that I think terrifies me yet excites me about the position in which I now find myself. I really want to make a positive difference at every stage, and sometimes fear inadvertently doing the opposite. The experience described in this account has taught me a lot about emergency medicine, and about how I react in an emergency situation in which I am asked to play an active role.

Reflective/ri'flektiv/concerned in reflection or thought; thoughtful, given to meditation

As I walk home my mind swims with thoughts. Rewind one hour. Sitting in the mess on take, talking with my PRHO about some benign matter. Her bleep goes and we are called to a ward (any ward, insignificant) to certify (a) death. It is the first time that I have been confronted with such a situation and I am not sure how I am going to react. Sure, I have been on a ward when a patient has died, but I have never, possibly through an unconscious avoidance, been present at certification, or seen a recently passed patient.

Death has been much talked about, but little can really prepare you for the reality. As we hurry up the innumerable stairs we discuss the formalities of death, the duty we have to play in a patient's passing. The curtain at the end of the bay is shut. We approach the nurses' station and are stopped; the gentleman's daughter is behind the curtains. We sit down and wait. In stark contrast to previous calls, there is no sense of pressure to complete the task. We fill the time with necessary paperwork with a hope to ease the process. The daughter leaves and, as she passes us, the nurses offer their condolences. There is no falseness about their words; everyone seems genuinely sad. In exchange the daughter replies with a warm smile and thanks for her father's care. The PRHO places her bleep on the desk and we walk to the bed. My mind is strangely empty of thoughts. As if an unspoken agreement has passed between us, we are silent as we enter the curtains. As passé as it sounds, the first thing I am hit by is the silence inside the curtains, in disparity with the busy hum of the ward. The PRHO silently goes about her duty:

> Fixed dilated pupils.
> No respiratory effort observed in three minutes.
> No pulse.
> No heart sounds for one minute.
> Death is certified.

We leave without a word passing between us and sit silently for a brief moment of contemplation, before I am asked if I am OK. I smile but don't feel yet able to answer the question.

Fast-forward and I'm walking again, and thinking about the episode. The first thing that I realise is that I am OK. I have often been frightened by my own emotions surrounding death, but now realise from talking to my PRHO that these are feelings that everyone has, and it is all right to feel like that. Second, I feel privileged. Privileged to have witnessed this process. Death in hospital is a common occurrence, an inevitable consequence of many disease processes, and as such becomes demystified, formalised even. Moreover in such an environment it can be easy to shelve dignity, yet throughout this episode I was constantly aware of conscious thought for its preservation.

We could have blundered behind the curtains, eager to complete a horrible task; we didn't and it was a conscious undertaking. Leaving the patient's daughter alone until she was ready seemed such a simple gesture, but it gave her a chance to say goodbye, to talk to her father or just to quietly think. Possibly she will remember that she was not hurried and be thankful for the time she was given.

The nurses' words were kind where they could so easily have been trite; the thought passes through my head that such kindness can only help to ease the pain of bereavement.

In leaving her bleep on the desk the PRHO performed another simple gesture that belied an underlying thoughtfulness. To be bleeped while certifying death would have somehow impoverished the manner in which the certification took place.

At the time I remember thinking that in an uncomfortable moment such as this it is all too easy to offer up some glib remark to disguise one's own discomfort. But the PRHO carried out the task silently and professionally. Indubitably the gravity of the certification, and the weight it carries, requires protocol, but as we stood behind the curtains, and as I walk, I realise the sensitivity with which the task can be carried out without compromising either dignity or the need for correctness, and it is a thought that stays with me.

As the whole process of shadowing ends and I write, it is without doubt that I have learned a great deal about the job of a PRHO. Becoming aware of the PRHO role has helped me gain confidence, and knowing my job will empower me to make it my own, within my own limitations.

But more importantly what shadowing has given me lies beyond learning objectives; it has given me the ability to confront the inevitable spectre of death, and the mindfulness to deal with death with the sensitivity and dignity it deserves; to know the right way to act, and to remember to pay every attention to the littlest details when dealing with death, for it is often the smallest gesture that sticks in people's minds.

Above all this experience is something that I am sure I will draw upon when confronted with similar experiences in my own career. Furthermore, writing this has enabled me to explicitly and introspectively explore and come to terms with my own feelings about death.

Shadowing – a challenge

My shadowing experience took place working with the cardiology team. Before I began, I was aware that working in such an environment was going to be a challenge in itself, let alone picking up all the useful hints on how to be a house officer. So, I tried to prepare myself for life as a cardiology PRHO.

However, day one as a shadow proved far more eventful than I could have imagined. It was all quite daunting at first. I walked straight into a CCU ward round and was asked if I'd like to note take. Despite being on the wards for a few years now, I hadn't really worked in such an intense environment. My first thought was 'Oh no, I can't remember my ECGs or the drugs used for heart failure!' But the experience was filling me with excitement for day one in August.

My main learning experience happened that afternoon – I chose it because it affected me most during the shadowing. One of the patients on CCU, an elderly gentleman, day three post-MI, really wasn't making any progress. Despite intensive treatment, he had failed to respond and was becoming visibly weaker. He had suffered three MIs in the past which had left his heart irreparably damaged. It became clear that should a further event occur, resuscitation would be inappropriate. As he was in and out of consciousness, it was decided that this decision should be discussed with the family first.

I was present at the discussion which was held in the relatives' room. Initially, the family wanted everything possible done, but eventually realised that to perform such invasive techniques would only put their father/husband through more suffering. The way this was handled by the SHO was exemplary, highlighting the need for good communication skills and sensitivity. Clearly, the family was upset but felt happy with the final decision. They believed that the patient should not be told about the DNAR order, as it would only cause him more distress.

Later that afternoon around 5 pm, just as the PRHO was looking forward to spending a rare hour in the sun, the alarm sounded and we all ran into CCU. It was our patient. He was in VT, barely conscious. With regards to the discussion earlier, it was decided that there was nothing more we could do and we all stood there watching, until he finally went into VF and passed away. My PRHO and I came back a while later to certify the death.

Clearly, this was a significant event needing reflection, so my PRHO suggested we took time out to debrief. Going over what had happened was really helpful, as I felt quite upset by the incident. I had found certifying the death eerie and unnerving, and the experience of someone dying before my eyes was something I'd not seen for quite some time. I thought how the family must feel.

There are many things I learned from that day, to name but a few – breaking bad news, the need for good communication skills, ethical dilemmas with regards to DNAR decisions, how to deal with an acutely ill patient, other clinical skills, certifying a death, dealing with difficult situations on an emotional level, and most importantly working together as a team. The death brought back personal memories for me and debriefing helped me to recognise these emotions and put them into context. Witnessing the events had taught me a lot, both practically and personally, about dealing with these patients and their families on a daily basis.

I identified some learning needs as a result: to improve my ECG interpretation (which I think I did!), know how to manage CCU patients post-MI, form filling and practicalities of the death of a patient, my role as a PRHO on the cardiology team, how to locate all equipment for cardiac arrests and methods of delivering bad news.

I have no doubt that my shadowing will benefit me as a PRHO, on many levels: from silly practicalities, like who's who, where things are on the ward, etc., to using the events I experienced as models on which to base my own methods of clinical practice. I hope I can break bad news as sensitively as my SHO did – obviously it's something we all dread doing, and much of it is down to experience, but this gave me some pointers on where to start.

At the beginning, I said I was prepared for a challenge. I gleaned more from my shadowing than I thought possible and it helped to allay some of the fears about starting in August. Rather than being daunted by the CCU, I am now looking forward to the experience. My PRHO was excellent and it was a shame she had leave booked for the second half. I can't wait to be part of the team in August and finally put my skills into practice. Just the small matter of some exams now …!

A difficult and perilous path

> Called to confirm death.
> No response to external stimuli.
> No pulse.
> No heart sounds for one minute.
> No breath sounds for three minutes.
> Pupils fixed and dilated.

This is a bleak start to any essay – hardly poetic in either sense of the word. How much more so must it be a bleak way for your death to be recorded? While it is, of course, both clinically important and legally necessary to confirm death, is this really a complete response to seeing a patient die?

It is often said by teachers that it is important to have a degree of emotional detachment when dealing with your patients and their loved ones. After all if we were to treat every death as the death of a member of our family we would soon lose the ability to cope with the job.

However, in busy hospital practice the balance all too often falls the other way. The balancing act between recognising patients as people and becoming too involved with the situation is a bit like being a child walking along the top of a wall at the edge of a cliff. It is a difficult and perilous path, and one that often slows your progress. You constantly risk toppling off the cliff and falling into the abyss of becoming too involved with the patients and their families and emotional burn-out. Would it not be easier to step off the wall and head directly across the flat land towards our ultimate goal?

Certainly this is what some doctors do and the reasons for this short cut are obvious. In order to treat our patients as people, in order to recognise their humanity, especially in this case, it is necessary, at least to some extent, to confront our own mortality. This takes a lot of time, emotional energy and courage, qualities that are all too often lacking at the end of a long shift and exhausting week.

But, while it may be tiring and is often difficult, it is necessary and important both for the patients and for the doctors. All too often there is little we can do with modern medicine to cure a disease, and palliation becomes important. At this point, our role as doctors should change. Palliative care is not just a matter of pain relief and muting of symptoms. While these things are obviously important, it is just as important to take the time to talk to the patient, to confront their worries and their fears, and time to talk to the relatives, to explain to them what has happened and what is likely to come.

We need to ask ourselves what we would consider important if we were in that position. By acknowledging the humanity and individuality of our patients, acknowledging the fact that they are not 'just' patients but are people as well, we not only give them a sense of worth and a reassuring ear, but we remind ourselves of why we are pursuing this career at all.

I would be the first to acknowledge that the pressures of the job make this a very idealistic situation. However, however little time you have as a doctor, and however senior you get, the necessity of just occasionally looking at your behaviour from the patient's perspective is still important. However good we become at surgery, or however talented a physician, if we, just once, treat our patient as a child because they have expressive dysphasia and cannot talk to us, or do not have time to explain why an operation is necessary, then we are not only not doing our jobs, but we are denying our patients the respect they are due.

For my own part, this acknowledgement of a patient's humanity is difficult and emotionally draining. However, if this shadowing course has taught me anything, it has made me realise how important, even as a junior, our time and effort is to patients, and how, ultimately, respecting their individuality, and helping them confront their mortality by looking into their eyes and confronting your own, makes you a far better doctor than efficiency with blood forms ever will. By giving the patients back their humanity every time we deal with the difficult situations that confront them, we become better at dealing with patients, and better at dealing with hard situations ourselves. If this essay emphasises anything it is that, while checking those pupil responses, it is important to look beyond that clinical test into that patient's eyes and acknowledge that one day that will be you. Perhaps that is why, as some recognition of this, those three final words are so important, both to the doctor and to the patient.

Rest in peace.

Failing to care is the worst sin of all

Medicine is all about saving lives – right? Finding new diagnoses and curing people of their ailments. Whether this is true or not, I believe it was what I thought. At my interview I am certain I had prepared an answer something to the effect of 'I want to study medicine to see science evolve in a dynamic way, to be on a continual learning curve and to combine a career in the world of science with an appreciation of art – the human body'. However, more importantly my true belief is that we all enter medicine in the belief that we are helping people; that we are going to relieve suffering and save lives. Throughout my five years in medicine I have undergone an immense personal and academic evolution. Partly this would happen anyway – five years is a long time and change is not surprising – but to study medicine it is necessary to grow up pretty quickly. Life on the wards exposes us to sights which the majority of the general public will never see, and emotional experiences for which on many occasions we are ill prepared. It is for this reason I think house officer shadowing and the experience of the fifth year of medical school is all important; with the experience of ward activities comes responsibility and an inability to escape from these experiences, but a need to attack them head on, however difficult they may seem. The exponential learning curve to which you sign up on accepting a place at medical school is one for which few of us, if any, had a true appreciation.

Life on the wards is variable; some days are quiet, but most provide challenges be they large or small. On occasion it is only moments into the day that we are faced with our most difficult scenarios. On a ward round one morning I was assisting the house officer by obtaining the observations, drug chart information and writing in the notes. As we approached one side room, I entered as previously, glancing to the bed to say good morning and then proceeded to pick up the nursing notes from the end of the bed. On receiving no reply I looked back to my patient, taking a more careful look. I could hear the team approaching, but for me it seemed time had suddenly stopped. My patient lay against the pillows, pale and fairly motionless. I wanted to believe he was just asleep and that I just needed to rouse him so that he would be ready to receive the entourage of the medical team. As I took his hand it was cold and clammy, but he was still breathing although laboured. It had been discussed previously that he should not be for resuscitation and as such I knew that calling the crash team was not an appropriate measure; however, more than anything else, I wanted to save this man and felt helpless with the knowledge that there wasn't anything practical I could do and no one I could call to do more. The team soon arrived and papers were signed, etc., to the effect that he should have no intervention and that the family should be informed. During this time my position near the bed had progressively been moved further back, I was in the back row now, lost for words but aware that while conversations ensued about how best to manage this man's affairs, no one was with him in his final moments, no one took his hand or spoke to him and I had to watch on in silence.

Personal experience is an amazing teacher. A year ago almost to this day, I sat with my Grandpa while he slipped away; it was the most traumatic experience of my life so far and yet I now view it as a privilege. To have shared his last moments and to have comforted him one last time is something for which I will be eternally grateful, safe in the knowledge that he wasn't alone. I am sorry that we could not show this man the same degree of compassion, that we couldn't provide him a family member or a friendly hand to hold. Medicine I realise now isn't about saving people – well, not always – it is about paving the way towards a comfortable future. All medicine is symptom relief; sometimes our palliation of symptoms can have curative intent and on other occasions we are unable to achieve this ultimate goal, but at no point should we consider an inability to cure a failing, but failing to care is the worst sin of all.

House officer shadowing taught me a multitude of things: how my job will work, what is expected of me and who is who in different departments, but more important than any of these more daily tasks of a house officer, it taught me that patients should never be forgotten and that we should support them until the end, because to forget our patients is to forget why we entered medicine in the first place.

Is there nothing else we can do?

The house job I shadowed was in oncology. Throughout my undergraduate training, I had encountered patients with cancer, usually in the context of surgical attachments. I had also witnessed medical professionals breaking bad news to anxious patients such as from histology reports or scan results. Although I realised that I would see cases of more advanced disease on the oncology wards, I thought that I was adequately prepared for my first week in the new hospital. Yet my confident attitude was not to last very long.

As I was working on the ward with my house officer and alongside the senior house officers, I was getting to know my patients a little better, especially those that were too unwell to be discharged immediately after treatment. One of my patients had developed a low urine output and a slight temperature while on antibiotics. I was asked to take blood cultures before starting intravenous antibiotics, and to insert a Foley catheter, which proved to be a difficult and hence not necessarily totally aseptic procedure. The patient had advanced oesophageal cancer. He had been admitted two weeks previously for insertion of a permanent central venous catheter for palliative chemotherapy, but he had not been well enough to undergo the procedure.

The next day, I found that he had been transferred into a side room of the ward because he had deteriorated and had become increasingly confused. His temperature was still elevated. There were more than the usual number of relatives by his bed. The house officer and I discussed with the patient's wife and his two sons that he was clearly dying and that comfort and palliation were now clinical priorities. The family agreed and expressed that they had been expecting the death of their father and husband since his admission to hospital. We started him on a palliative syringe driver, and discontinued fluids and antibiotics.

All the time, I found myself wondering if we could not offer this gentleman anything else to improve his condition. I also contemplated about the reason for the patient's elevated temperature and was eager for the culture results to come back. Perhaps we should also send a catheter urine specimen for culture? What if my poor catheter insertion technique was to blame for the patient's condition? Why could we not give the antibiotics another day or two to work and bring the temperature down?

Eventually he died, later that afternoon, surrounded by his family. At the end of the day, it occurred that all ward doctors and a couple of nurses looking after him were meeting in the doctors' office. His death naturally became the main topic of our conversation, and I was able to voice my thoughts. It emerged that the nurses had been concerned since his admission and found the doctors' plan for an invasive procedure inappropriate. They appeared relieved when it was recognised that he was not going to improve again. The senior house officer admitted that it often takes too long to switch from medical to palliative mode in cancer patients, because doctors often did not have time to look at the whole patient.

In hindsight, I agree. I think that the attitude of most doctors, especially hospital doctors, is interventional rather than reflective. We order many investigations and treatments in a reflex to numbers and individual parameters rather than the patient's clinical needs. In the vast majority of cases, blood cultures and insertion of a urinary catheter in response to a raised temperature and low urine output seem perfectly acceptable. However, the ground is more slippery in patients with cancer. The decision-making process for any intervention needs to be more painstaking and patients' wishes must be taken into account. The ethical principles of beneficence as well as non-maleficence and especially of autonomy come to mind.

I was feeling somewhat guilty that we could not offer the patient any more treatment. However, nobody expected more treatment for him; they hoped that we would stop intervening. His family had anticipated his death, and they simply wanted peace and comfort for him during his last hours. I felt the burden of guilt and worry taken from my shoulders, and recognised that death does not equal failure of treatment. Moreover, I wished that we had communicated better with the nurses about our patient. Our informal debriefing session proved a good opportunity, but perhaps it was a little late.

Just as I was going to leave the oncology block together with the house officer, one of the patient's sons came up to thank us for everything we had done that day. And on the way out of the hospital, the house officer reassured me about my catheter insertion technique. She had observed me through a gap in the curtains.

Clearing up

I'm too hot.

But the air in this room is still and cold, the atmosphere is brittle and tense, and expectation hovers around my head. Nervous panic prickles through me; I am on my own. I force myself to look at the pale face next to me, eyes staring blankly. I have to look away. Nothing prepares you for this. I don't feel ready and I don't know what to do. I try to focus on what the Coroner is saying; he is sensible and calm, I should listen, but I look out the window and try to forget where I am. I can't. He has finished speaking. The others in the room clap in apprehensive appreciation. The shadowing introduction is over and they are turning us loose. It's time to meet our fate.

My period of job shadowing took place, fairly uniquely I believe, on an oncology unit. Maybe it is for this reason that the lasting impressions I took from it concerned the end of life. I think it is underestimated how unprepared students feel on the first day. I was terrified somebody would ask me to do something beyond my capabilities, I thought the job would involve skills and knowledge far superior to mine, and I'm not sure that feeling ever left me over the two weeks. I will briefly describe two incidents that were particularly memorable, in very contrasting ways.

Nobody died on my first day. The patients we saw were fairly well, often with complex social circumstances, in for some minor treatments and waiting for discharge. One lady chatted in a thick Irish accent about her eight children as she inhaled heavily on her oxygen. She showed me the stones from her husband's grave that she had taped to her hand so as never to lose them, and begged me to tell her son that she was required to rest, as she didn't want to speak with him. Despite her wasted face her eyes still twinkled and although she spoke of having had her time, she was desperate to go home for just a little while before the end. She achieved her final wish, but after less than 24 hours she returned, very ill, having rapidly deteriorated. She was delirious and agitated until she was sedated, and died not altogether peacefully the next day. The relatives were distraught. One daughter sat outside weeping, and it was hours before my PRHO and I could go in to certify the death.

I know I am lucky to come from a background not yet touched by the death of a loved one. I sit safe in my cocoon of health and feel grateful for the fortune I am blessed with. Death was in another world I hadn't encountered yet, incredibly not even in medical school. Perhaps this made me even less prepared. I was moved when we entered the room and she lay there, perfectly motionless, still clutching the precious stones. I was disturbed that there were still noises when we listened to her chest and I felt guilty for intruding on such a private moment for all concerned. It was a difficult experience, made more poignant by the youngest daughter's tearful request for reassurance that she really had passed on, as her mother had been scared of being buried alive.

When it next happened, it didn't move me as much, and eventually, in a short space of time, it became just another part of the job. We shouldn't grieve over every patient surely, but I was shocked at the speed with which I and everyone around me isolated themselves from the human emotions and carried on.

Later that week we were asked to see a gentleman who was receiving treatment for bone metastases which had been fairly successful. His wife was concerned about him, as he had spoken to the consultant earlier and believed that he had been told he was cured. On meeting him he was alert and cheerful, his cheeks were flushed and he greeted us eagerly. We asked him what his understanding of the situation was and he told us how happy he was that he was cured. The house officer very carefully and kindly explained that this was not so. I watched the light drain from his eyes as he lost his future for a second time. His head bowed and his weariness returned to his face. He almost pleaded that we would never give up on treating him. His hope was the only thing he had left. His wife blinked back tears and squeezed his arm as the promise was made, in a conversation that should never have taken place.

Anybody can go on the endless ward round that is a PRHO's job and somehow manage blood bottles, drugs charts and clerking. It requires a set of skills that is surprisingly removed from those experienced in medical school. What makes the role unique is the difference made by the sensitive handling of people, good communication, and never losing sight of the human emotions in every case.

Death and social death

Bizarrely, in five years of medical training having patients die is not something that I spent much time considering. The medicine we are taught is focused on how to cure sickness and evade death. My shadowing experience wasn't. It was as much to do with managing the dying. Perhaps this experience was down to the nature of the ward I was on, a Care of the Elderly ward. Or perhaps it is an accurate representation of hospital medicine, and as much as we'd like to think that hospitals are places where people's lives are saved, they are in fact really just as much places where people come to die. In *Madness and Civilisation* Foucault talks about the 'Great Confinement' where the mentally ill in France become institutionalised. An 'out-of-sight, out-of-mind' mentality prevails. In a sense this has become true of death in contemporary Western society. Death has been taken out of the home and institutionalised in hospitals.

Almost the first thing I was involved with was to go to the morgue in order to fill out a death certificate. A great deal of time was spent re-reading the patient's notes, considering how to fill out the parts of the death certificate, completing the paperwork in general. The examination of the body was perfunctory. A glance at the wrist band to confirm identity rather than lingering on the dead woman's face. A wave of a metal detector over the chest, eliminating the chance of a pace maker, rather than a touching of the corpse. Then quickly back to fill out the cremation form as well. The next week, there would be more forms to fill for a different patient. This time a patient whom I'd taken blood from, talked to on ward rounds, in short a patient I knew. The process was of course the same, a lingering over the forms, a fly-by of the corpse and back to the forms. Engaging with the paperwork served to avoid engaging with the death of the person. A line was drawn under the incident and we moved on. Not necessarily a vicious approach, but far from virtuous. Morally acceptable, rather than morally ideal.

The next incident that impressed itself upon me was that of having a patient for whom very little could be done. This particular patient was in obvious distress. She called out over and over again complaining of nausea. She had been on the ward for months and had been seen by a number of specialists, including the palliative care team, all to no avail. This patient was too ill to go to a nursing home and too well to die. However, the feeling of the team was that nothing further could be done, and that decision had a powerful effect. In the eyes of the medical team the patient had already died a 'social death'. Physical death was simply a formality to be awaited. In effect a barrier was placed between the patient and the staff. The effect of the barrier was to distance that patient, although I don't suppose her medical – as opposed to psychological or spiritual – care was adversely effected, in order to reduce our need to contemplate the nature of mortality.

The reasons why these incidents seemed significant to me may say more about my personal reflections on mortality (in general, of my own and of that of those dear to me) than I suppose it does of the actual patients involved. In retrospect, I do think it is a little fantastical that I've got so far as a medical student without really dealing with dying patients. This realisation has been reinforced by the palliative care block – which I am just doing at the moment – where the concentration of 'dying' patients has been greater than ever before.

These collected experiences may lead to the following changes in my approach to my medical career. I am now more conscious than before of the futility of a lot of medicine, and am in a sense happier to accept there are occasions where nothing more can be done. And there is also the realisation that talking about a person's impending death to that person is one of the trickiest, squirm-inducing conversations anyone is ever likely to have. I am hoping they get easier.

There is nothing more we could have done

At first I thought the aims of the shadowing experience were to become familiar with the practicalities of being a house officer, such as which computer systems they use, how to order x-rays and where the doctors' mess is. However, I soon learned that the time spent exclusively with the house officer you were shadowing had the added benefit of teaching one so much more about what it means to be a doctor. Witnessing interactions with different patients in different situations, as well as experiencing how it feels to be in charge of patient care, taught me a lot more than how to fill in radiology forms and keep up with ward rounds. If this all sounds a little vague, here is a brief account of one of the turning moments in my transition from medical student to imminent house officer.

I was shadowing a friendly, extremely competent surgical house officer. We were on call that day, and so admitted surgical patients from A&E as well as covering the wards until 10 pm. Earlier in the day one of the patients, a 60-year-old lady, had suffered a 'funny turn'. She had had a laparotomy for a cholecystectomy over six weeks ago and had been admitted a few days previously due to severe right upper quadrant pain. This was thought to be due to gallstones, and she was expected to have an ERCP the following day.

The episode earlier in the day involved her feeling very dizzy and faint and, although she didn't lose consciousness, her blood pressure became undetectable, she was pale and her pulse became weak and bradycardic. Luckily a senior anaesthetist happened to be on the ward and quickly assisted, raising the foot of her bed, initialising fluids and administering a small amount of atropine. The patient seemed to recover and her blood pressure improved to about 110/70 (it had previously been around 140 systolic). The patient admitted that similar episodes had happened recently, where she experienced severe upper quadrant pain followed by a feeling of dizziness when she became pale and often had to sit or lie down for a period of time. It was concluded that she had suffered from a vasovagal faint in response to her pain and was given more fluids as it was noted her urine output had been poor for most of the day.

At around 6 pm the nurses were concerned and asked the on-call house officer (us) to review this lady. A thorough history was taken and a similar conclusion was reached; the lady claimed she felt much better, a little 'woozy' but thought that was also due to the morphine she had been given for the pain. The patient was alert, communicating well and, although her systolic blood pressure was still wavering at 100–110 mmHg, she did not seem a patient to be very concerned about. It was decided that we would ask the SHO on call to review her during the evening just in case.

A few hours later we were bleeped again as the lady's systolic blood pressure had dropped again slightly to 90 mmHg systolic. It was decided the SHO should review her immediately. Blood was taken and although her Hb was low (8.9, compared to 11.7 the day before), this was thought to be dilutional due to the fluids she had been given. The lady was reviewed again at 1 am by a different SHO, in a similar state, and again bloods were taken; however, when the registrar saw her at 3 am that morning, her blood pressure had dropped to 80/50 and her Hb was 3.5. She was immediately taken to theatre where it transpired that she had actually been leaking blood from around her porta hepatis and had collected over 8 litres of blood in her abdominal cavity. Despite being transfused huge amounts of blood constituents, the patient only managed to hold on until noon the next day, when, in ITU, it became apparent that she would not recover from such a huge insult.

This unfortunate story could be used to show the importance of recognising a falling blood pressure as an important clinical sign and the fact that if an individual suffers from a simple vaso-vagal event, their blood pressure should recover quickly and completely. It could also be used to highlight that despite a convincing story, such as the history given by the patient of having similar dizzy episodes following the bouts of pain, one should not immediately accept diagnoses of exclusion as fact until other more serious ones have been disproved. One could even criticise the care of this patient prior to when she fainted earlier in the day, by questioning why an ultrasound had not been performed to prove the presence of gallstones, instead of just waiting for her ERCP. However, I think this story also helps demonstrate another, much more important point.

When my house officer discovered what had happened as she came into work the next morning her reaction was typical of any compassionate person. Her initial reaction was to go down to ITU to check on the lady's progress, and despite being obviously affected by the poor prognosis, she went back to the ward to start the day. It wasn't until the ward sister said a simple comment along the lines of 'It was terrible what happened, but there is nothing more we could have done' that the house officer, overcome with emotion, started to cry.

Medicine is a strange profession. In the past it used to be seen as helping people through sickness, perhaps preventing death where possible by supporting symptoms, controlling pain and providing nutrition and medications. As time goes on and medical advances become more sophisticated, the view is sometimes that when patients die it is not because of something that naturally happens, but is a fault of the medical team. True, sometimes people are to blame, but then at other times things are unexpected, such as this case. It was still unknown where the blood had come from; however, reactive haemorrhage six weeks after an operation is extremely rare, and perhaps one would be forgiven for not considering it initially. Also, the house officer had done all that was in her control, she had alerted her senior when she was concerned, and four other people had reviewed the patient before the decision for surgery was made.

Sometimes so much emphasis is put on the practicalities of becoming a doctor that as students you can forget about the emotional side of it. The job itself is stressful but when you add in the fact that you are working in a very precious area of life, the preserving or letting go of it, where patients and their relatives are often experiencing many challenging situations, you can see how easy it is to lose control. Perhaps that's the real lesson here: sometimes things aren't in your control, and it's through no fault of your own, but if you do your best and recognise when you need to talk to someone then you are already one step ahead.

Why are we doing what we do?

We were on take that night; my house officer and I were covering the wards with the odd jobs that always seem to need doing when we were bleeped by one of the wards. Apparently the daughter of one of the inpatients was very worried that her mother had suddenly become very quiet and unresponsive. Her mother had not arrested but according to the nurse on the 'phone the daughter was becoming increasingly loud, and demanding that a doctor see her mother. We were told that the sons of the same patient had arrived as well and wanted to know the current situation. The nurse on the end of the 'phone was quite adamant that we go and deal with the relatives. Telling me that in situations like this he didn't have much choice my house officer agreed to go immediately.

When we entered the ward, we were accosted by two of the sons who more or less led us into the side room where their mother was. Present in the room was also the daughter, another brother and their father. I felt a bit overwhelmed and outnumbered at the situation but my house officer politely asked the family to leave so that he could examine the patient. They were reluctant, but he said that the room was too small for all of them and that he would see them immediately afterwards in the day room. When they filed out he whispered to me to go get the patient's notes, as she wasn't one of his patients and we needed to know what the ongoing situation was. Reading through the notes we discovered that the lady had just developed renal failure and would have to have dialysis. It was the opinion of the renal physicians that this would be too much for her frail health and they thought that a Do Not Attempt Resuscitation note should be discussed with the family and put into her notes.

This would be the first time my house officer had to do this and he was understandably worried about how to broach this subject, especially with such an aggressive family. I asked him whether he could ask the SHO but he said there would be little chance there. He felt that the SHO would not support him or even offer to help. He was always doing his job and didn't really care about any problems my house officer might have. We were effectively on our own.

Examining the patient we found that she hadn't suffered a stroke but her condition had deteriorated. We had to relay this to the family as well as to discuss the DNAR. It was uncomfortable for us as we walked into the day room with all eyes upon us. He told them our findings regarding her deterioration in health and that the next few days would be very hard on their mother. He didn't directly mention the subject of the DNAR until one of the brothers asked about it. It was a difficult situation all round; how the decision was reached in the end was another matter irrelevant to this account, but the decision to not attempt resuscitation in the event of a further decline in health was agreed upon.

Why did I choose this incident? It was because of the dynamics of the situation, an aggressive family, an unsupportive senior, feeling tired and out of one's depth but still having to do your job, and praying that it doesn't go horribly wrong. Each of these on its own would be daunting enough during your house jobs but all of them together was really frightening. Who could we have asked for help? It was late at night, everyone was busy, we were tired and had few ideas. I believe that because I was there the nurse did not offer to accompany the house officer to talk to the family.

Thankfully it went well; by first going into how much the family were aware of their mother's health we had a foundation to build upon. Being honest, empathic and, foremost of all, not being too doctor-like saw us through this situation. I learned that by involving the family in their mother's care, with a simple explanation of the situation, they effectively made the decision themselves.

It is only when we realise that it isn't about doing all that is possible, but why we are doing it, that we can learn from one experience to the next. People skills are one of the most important aspects of this future job, not just within your team, your ward or your patients. For whatever reason, my house officer didn't have the best relationship with his SHO and felt he had to do things on his own most of the time. I don't know whose fault this was, or if there was any fault, but effective relations make effective teams. Regarding the family, I believe they felt that before this night, they weren't given any information regarding their mother. The nurses told them that a doctor would talk to them; the doctor who saw the lady previously did not wish to discuss DNAR with the family and left it to the next person. My house officer was that next person, and, although uncomfortable, through sharing the problem with the family, he forged a relationship with them and all agreed that DNAR was what was best for their mother.

It is often forgotten that patients aren't 'the lady with renal failure', 'the guy with the hernia', or someone with good signs. The lady in bed 12 is someone's friend, someone's wife and someone's mother.

What if this was my mother?

What would I want to know?

How would I react?

What would make me happy with her care?

These are all questions I think we should ask ourselves whenever we meet the family of any of the people in our care. I know these are the questions I will ask myself when someone says to me … 'Isn't the daughter/son/husband/wife/patient really annoying?'

Is it our treatment of them that is doing the annoying?

Certification of death

Thursday mornings are consultant ward rounds. So we, the firm, set off circling the hospital and descending on wards, so that we can visit our patients and offer them a few words of reassurance.

After a few hours my feet start to ache, my stomach starts to rumble and my brain is having difficulty recalling all the names, clinical details and lab results. All the patients begin to merge into one another and I start to realise that to be a good PRHO I am somehow going to have to expand my memory.

We enter a new ward and collect the notes before going to see the next patient. I recognise her; she is the lady with aortic regurgitation that we had teaching on a week ago. It is usually difficult to communicate with her, as she is very deaf and has left her hearing aid at home, but today she is quite quiet. Her pulmonary oedema has got a bit worse and she has sacral oedema. We discuss the plan – our registrar thinks we should catheterise her to monitor her fluid output, and our consultant thinks we should contact her relatives regarding DNAR status. We then move on and finish the ward round before going for a well-earned coffee.

During our break a nurse comes in. She has some bad news. The lady we have just seen has died. I am shocked. Why did I not realise she was so close to death?

The PRHO that I am shadowing asks if I would like to do the certification. I agree. I've seen it done before so I know what to do – besides, it will be my job to do it in August.

We go up the ward and ominously make our way across to the side room. As we enter, I immediately notice an aura of quietness and stillness, as if we have shut the whole world out.

I approach the bed feeling uneasy, as I cannot launch into my usual introduction and spiel about being a medical student. I stand there for what seems like ages, trying to compose myself. It isn't as if I haven't seen a dead body before, I've seen plenty in the dissecting room and on the wards, but it is different actually having to touch someone so freshly dead.

I finally manage to pull myself together and using my pen-torch I check if her pupils are fixed and dilated. They are. It feels like looking in to an abyss. I go on to check the pulses, which are absent, and I then listen to the chest. Listening to nothing feels odd, your mind plays tricks on you, you hear your own heart beat thumping in your ears and any slight movement of the stethoscope creates a sound resembling a breath. I listen for three minutes, although it feels a lot longer, and still I hear nothing. I have now finished and I am convinced that she is dead, but in the back of my mind I still expect her to speak or move, or do something. I close her eyes and we leave, having completed the last service that we can ever do for her.

I chose this case as I thought that it raised several important issues. First, it concerned me that I hadn't recognised earlier that this patient was dying. Having now completed the palliative care part of the course, I feel that I would be in a better position to identify patients in the terminal phase of their illness. However, when you are involved in a patient's care, I think that it can be hard to step back and appreciate that they are slowly deteriorating.

Second, I was surprised at how hard I found it to deal with a dead person. I thought that I was well prepared, so I was shocked by how much I was affected by it. This is perhaps an example of our vulnerability as doctors and highlights the need for good self-care.

This case also helped me to reflect on the fact that dealing with death is a huge part of our job and it carries with it a huge responsibility. We are told from day one that being a doctor is not about curing everyone, and that, in reality, good end-of-life care can be one of the things that our patients and relatives appreciate the most.

This case also raises several ethical issues such as the timing and the way in which DNAR orders are discussed with relatives. In this case, it could perhaps have been discussed with the relatives at a better time, but is there ever a good time? Another question which it raised was how aggressive our medical interventions should be so close to death. This lady had been catheterised earlier that morning, which could be viewed as having been unnecessary.

I think that this experience has benefited me in many ways. It has improved my practical skills in terms of dealing with death, but it has also prepared me psychologically. I now think that I will be far less daunted when I begin my job in August, and I am very grateful to my house officer for giving me that confidence. I also think that it has made me aware of the importance of sometimes stepping back, to get a true picture of what is going on.

Fast bleep to ward one

The sun streamed through the windows of the hospital. Outside, the city basked in the glory of a sunny spring day, daffodils bobbing their yellow heads in the breeze. Inside, the Care of the Elderly ward round reached the next bed, the locker crowded with cards and bunches of flowers.

It had been a long morning – I had spent the last three hours on a mammoth ward round, taking us the length and breadth of the hospital. I could feel a faint pang of hunger in my stomach and my concentration slipped from the ward round discussion to thoughts of summer and finishing exams. The house officer beside me also seemed to be finding it hard to concentrate, but we were both dragged abruptly back to reality by the harsh sound of his bleep ... 'fast bleep to Ward One' ... 'fast bleep to Ward One' ... the house officer sprang into action and began running down the ward, as I hurried along behind. We ran down the corridor, my stethoscope swinging violently round my neck, and across to the other side of the hospital, people standing aside to let us pass. A minute later we rounded the corner into ward one and arrived panting at the nurses' desk. My heart pounded with fear, unsure what to expect. One of the patients was fitting. We hurried to his bed, around which the curtains had been hastily drawn.

He was 75 and had widespread malignancy. He had been admitted with a haemoglobin of 5 and had been transfused. I first met him the previous day and warmed to him immediately. He had been sitting up in bed, smiling and chatting, thanking the doctors profusely for making him feel so much better and introducing us to his relatives. There had been talk of when he could leave hospital and despite his poor prognosis, which he fully understood, I had been amazed at how cheerful and positive he was.

By the time we arrived he had stopped fitting, but I was shocked at the contrast between the previous day and now. He looked moribund, was barely conscious and breathing rapidly into an oxygen mask. He was incontinent of urine and red blood seeped into the stark white sheet from where his cannula had come out. As I stood at the foot of the bed, the familiar feelings I have often experienced as a medical student began to creep in. I have never been the most pushy of medical students and often feel like I'm in the way, that I'm just not useful and wish I could shrink to fit as small a space as possible, an art which still eludes me despite having had five years of practice! However, this time it was different – I was going to be doing this job in less than six months and I was acutely aware that I should be able to deal with such a situation.

Obviously having similar thoughts, the house officer turned and asked me what I thought he should do. With visions of my lecturer pacing animatedly up and down the front of level nine lecture theatre, I went through ABC and was heartened to find the house officer nodding in agreement. After making sure he was comfortable, prescribing diazepam and writing in the notes, we were asked to see his relatives, who had just arrived after being called to say he had taken a turn for the worse.

The house officer explained the situation in a gentle and compassionate way to the concerned relatives, who were naturally upset and wanted to know what was going on. I watched as he dealt sensitively and yet honestly with their questions, taking time to check they had understood.

During shadowing, I spent much of my time getting to grips with the basics – the layout of wards, using the computers, etc. However, events such as that described above made me realise exactly what roles and responsibilities I will have. Anyone can look up blood results and write forms but not everyone knows what to do when faced with an ill person who requires your care. It was a turning point when I realised that, yes, finals permitting, it would be me doing the job in five months time, and that, yes, despite all my doubts, I could actually do it.

Seeing the house officer deal with relatives also made me realise what an important link house officers can be and how important good communication skills are. It would have been easy for him to rush off to rejoin the ward round and catch up with his jobs. However, it was nice to see him make the time to talk to the relatives and treat them in such a considerate and respectful manner. I am sure at times next year I will feel I am only employed to do mundane, sometimes boring, jobs, but as the house officer I will get to know the patients and relatives well, often better than other members of my team. To be a good house officer, in the eyes of other doctors, you have to be organised and efficient but I think patients and their relatives are also looking for something more. They want to be made better but they also want to be treated as people. By remembering to do simple things, such as talking to them, giving them time despite being busy, I think a good house officer in the eyes of other doctors can be an excellent house officer in the eyes of the patient.

The patient didn't really regain full consciousness again. He was spared further blood tests and spent his last days with his relatives, who had been prepared that the end was near. In the end, he passed away peacefully with his wife at his side two days after we were called to see him.

Looking after patients at the end of their lives is something I will get used to. As a doctor we want to make people better and it can be tempting to continue with investigations and vigorous treatment. However, difficult though it may be to do nothing, there are times when we will be required to stand back and let nature take its course.

I am sure there will be many more patients like the gentleman described in my career and many difficult situations that I will have to handle but I hope that the lessons I learned during my shadowing will stay with me and help me to remember what a special job we do as doctors.

The event

I bleeped my house officer to find out what she was up to, having been on medical on call all weekend. I had agreed to join her for Sunday evening to get a taster for what it would be like. 'I think you should come to the ward straight away; it would be a good learning experience for you.' I arrived to find her in apron and gloves clutching bags of saline, in a side room trying to resuscitate an elderly gentleman who was having a PR bleed. She had been there for the last half an hour on her own with the nurses, and had managed to just about stabilise him. He was still bleeding profusely and was clearly very sick, and in need of an operation.

This elderly gentleman had no previous history of gastrointestinal problems. He had suddenly had a small bleed in the morning, and so she had called the surgical team for some advice, but was told to watch and wait. Then just after lunch he started to bleed severely so she had been called back.

Within the space of an hour after me arriving, the medical registrar arrived and decided, having spoken to the nurses, that he was capable of having some sort of surgical procedure to try and stop the bleeding. The surgical team appeared, first the SHO, then the registrar and then finally the consultant. From ITU appeared the anaesthetist registrar on call. Eventually the medical consultant on call was tracked down in the local supermarket and was called in.

It was finally decided after a lot of discussion not to take him to theatre, to stop transfusing him, and to make him as comfortable as possible, giving him only what fluid was still up and running. The family had been waiting outside the room all this time being plied with tea by the nurses. They were finally allowed to come in to say their goodbyes, and the teams dispersed. He died early the next morning.

I chose this event because it stood out so much during my fortnight shadowing. It was an opportunity to see ethics 'in action' as a debate evolved around me – the difference being that this ethical debate was about someone dying in the next room, so people could not spend hours discussing the issues extensively. The whole situation boiled down to the surgeons not wanting to operate, but reluctantly so, because of how he was before this episode. The medics wanted the surgeons to at least try something, for example a gastroscopy to see if he was bleeding from varices. The PRHO and the nurses who had been with him from the start all wanted the surgeons to try anything. As for the family outside the door, well …

So, do the surgeons operate on this man, who is elderly and might not even survive the anaesthetic, but who had a good quality of life before this episode? They decided not to, and went against the wishes of everyone else around them. I felt that this must have been a hard decision, but at the end of the day it would be them who would be operating and taking over his care. They made sure that everyone agreed or at least understood why they had made that decision, including the nurses. The medics felt helpless as they were not in a position to do anything apart from giving him more blood, which the haematology department were getting irritated about, apparently seeing it as 'wasted materials'. The nurses who had known the man before any of this had happened were understandably very upset but realised why the surgeons had made their decision.

The mood on the ward once the surgeons had left was subdued; I think many people felt let down. The consultant surgeon had gone to speak to the relatives so they fully understood the situation, but the medics and nurses were left to decide what they could do, if anything. It was then decided to stop all treatment, to try not to prolong the inevitable that was becoming distressing for everyone. The consultant medic, who I think is rarely called in on a weekend when he is on call, made one last-ditch attempt to get the surgeons to try a gastroscopy, knowing that they would say no, but it made everyone else feel that they really had done everything possible.

This really was an impossible situation with everyone left feeling as if they could have done more. What really struck me was how the PRHO handled the entire situation. She supported the nurses who were on the 'front line', liaised with the rest of her team, and called them at appropriate times. She chose not to speak to the relatives as she realised she was out of her depth, and so asked her consultant to speak to them. She called the surgical team early so that they were aware of the patient. All of that, while continuing to keep the patient alive while the decisions were being made, supporting me, and keeping me up to date with everything. I think in this sort of situation you do just need to hold everything together and she was a great example, and I can only hope that in the same situation, I will handle it with the same calmness and maturity that she did.

My first crash call!

Let me set the scene … My first day shadowing – keen and enthusiastic as we all were – rocked up to the ward, stethoscope round my neck, pockets bulging with pens, tourniquet, maglite and other essential items, cheese and onion in one hand, shoes polished, shirt ironed, clean shaven and raring to make a good impression. Met the team, who were very friendly and keen to get me involved as soon as possible. It was fortunate that the PRHO I was shadowing was actually a close friend of mine, which made the awkwardness you occasionally get when starting on a new firm less apparent. This also eased my way into getting on the right side of the multitude of nurses on the ward (the odd beverage put their way also helped!). And so I got started.

For the first day I was told to observe how the ward was run – where the blood forms went, when the phlebotomists came round, how to get results from the computer, etc. I followed my PRHO around like a hawk during the ward round, examining every single miniscule aspect of the job, asking the most obvious questions and generally trying to get a grip of the job. It was strange to think that these PRHOs have only been doing the job for just over six months and yet they seem so proficient and knowledgeable. I wonder first where they have gained all these skills and second whether I will ever be as proficient … scary thought!

Then … halfway through the round a buzzer goes off on the ward. I don't think much of it, nor does the PRHO who indicates that one of the patients has probably pressed the alarm button in the bathroom. A nurse then rushes up to us in a fluster saying that one of the patients has collapsed while getting out of the bath. My heart rate goes wild … I become excited and scared at the same time … a million and one things are dashing through my mind – is this an arrest? If so, what do I do? What happens if they ask me to do something and I get it wrong? What happens if he dies? I am suddenly reassured by the fact that the PRHO and SHO are both standing next to me and I suddenly think 'Oh, it's OK, some proper doctors are here, they'll know what to do'. Both the PRHO and SHO are looking calm and sauntering towards the bathroom in question. It suddenly dawns on me that in five months time it could be me in the same situation … would I be acting so calmly … I very much doubt it!

We got to the bathroom. The elderly man (who was not one of our patients) was sitting in a wheelchair; he was pale and didn't look to be breathing. The SHO examined him quickly and the man was shallow breathing and had a weak carotid pulse. We quickly transferred him to his bed, which was nearby, and laid him down flat. The SHO took control and calmly asked the nurses to bring out and set up all the monitoring equipment and to bring the defibrillator. He didn't ask me to do anything so I just stood there and watched, and basically felt a bit useless. The patient's heart rate was getting slower and weaker and the patient started 'Cheyne-Stoking'; the crash call was made. The SHO and PRHO still remained calm and clinical, even though this was a critical situation. Basic life support had started when the paddles of the defibrillator were ready to be placed on the patient. The rhythm showed VF and so he shocked it. By this time the cubicle filled with people all huffing and puffing, ready for action … the crash team. They took over in a similarly calm and methodical manner. IV access was gained, relevant drugs were administered, airway and breathing were maintained and shockable rhythms were shocked; however, the patient did not pull through.

For me, to see someone arresting right in front of me was a shock. Various emotions came over me – panic, confusion, uselessness. I have been to arrest calls before but had never been there at the beginning. It all seemed to happen so quickly. How would I cope on my own in such a situation? I guess I started to question my ability to perform in emergency situations. How do you deal with it afterwards? The crash team left and the SHO carried on with the ward round as if nothing had happened – do we become desensitised?

I have recently done the ILS course and therefore feel reasonably confident in my ability to function in emergency situations, and therefore this part of the course has been invaluable. It has also been taught during ethics and communication skills how to cope with stress and grief, and how important it is to talk to others (close colleagues and friends) to help you through it.

This event has taught me two key points. First, try not to question your own ability in these situations, act calmly and methodically and do your best for the patient – you might be their only hope. Second, as doctors we are faced with death on a regular basis; this does not mean we are impervious to normal human characteristics such as grief and sorrow. We should therefore confront these emotions and take time out to deal with them. This has been an extremely useful learning experience that I think will benefit every aspect of my PRHO job.

Feeling the fear

'Bye-bye Dr David' were the last words that I heard from the patient as I walked away after doing one of my perfunctory examinations. The next morning as I was swept up in the slipstream of the cardiology ward round we were stopped abruptly by meeting his wife and son who had just been to view his body. Condolences were given and the team was thanked (which I still find quite strange, even now). The ward round continued on, but not quite such apace.

The patient was in his mid-eighties and had suffered from heart failure for a number of years and it was this that had necessitated his admission. Unfortunately just as it had seemed his heart failure was being brought under control, he had contracted pneumonia. This put further strain on his heart and he had been deteriorating despite optimum treatment. He and his family had been told that the situation was now very serious indeed and they had decided against resuscitation.

When I examined him the day before he was patently unwell, but he did not strike me as pre-morbid. Yet when I saw his wife and son (who I hadn't met) coming towards us, I knew that he must have died.

I was struck in two ways. Initially it was the not yet familiar reinforcement of the finality and permanence of death, at least in this life, reminding me of the incredibly precarious thread wire we walk and how precious it is, but this feeling isn't new and I've encountered it since I did work experience in a hospice to spruce up my CV. I've come across it lots of times as an undergraduate but not so many as to become inured to it. The second feeling and one that I hadn't really come across before was 'The Fear'.

To clarify, this is different from the fear which surrounds finals that stalks all fifth years on their descent into them. That fear pushes us to learn esoteric syndromes, spread rumours like the Hanta virus, and infuse our language with the constant drip-drip of medical terminology.

The fear I feel won't disappear after the final 'Stop writing please'. Nor will any amount of Dionysian excess eliminate it. The fear isn't about exams, but the job itself. How would I have coped if Mr R recovered from his pneumonia but was destined to come to the ward on 3 August and deteriorate then? This was the fear I felt.

Part of the reason I wanted (and want) to become a doctor was the responsibility of making important life and death decisions, the adrenaline of sirens and blue lights. This of course is fine in a detached, armchair sort of way, but when it is actually you carrying the badge, bleep and burden, then it starts to appear a lot less glamorous and a lot more frightening. Because this is real life with real people, not a part of my generalised 18 year old's idea of 'doctoring'.

The fear partly arises from how I will feel when I make the first important error. This is going to happen certainly within the first few months, when something I forgot to do wasn't checked up on and a patient's clinical outcome is adversely affected. The god-awful feeling of guilt that will sweep over me as the realisation sinks in is gut-wrenching. There is nothing I can do to prevent this happening, although I can try and minimise these mistakes as much as possible. We are of course human and it is human to err but the responsibility and guilt I will feel will be quite overwhelming. It is the fear of letting those down who have put themselves in your care. That duty or onus or burden of care can sometimes be immense.

To read so far would be to paint a picture of someone who is totally petrified of the beginning of August, whereas nothing could be further from the truth. I am exhilarated by the prospect of walking onto 'my' ward with 'my patients'. Finally, getting the responsibility after six years. I really can't wait. But that does not mean in some situations I will not be very scared. The story in vogue at the moment is of a newly qualified PRHO answering her crash bleep and being the first doctor to arrive at the ward. The sister spies her and shouts 'Move back, the doctor's here', to which the relieved PRHO says 'Oh thank God!' and looks behind her. The vast majority of the fifth year can empathise completely.

However, as a house officer often there is a lot more back-up in the shape of SHOs, nurses and more senior members of the team. A large proportion of my time will be spent filling out forms, doing and chasing bloods and battling with the obstreperous veins of the town's population. The sort of incidents I'm apprehensive about encountering early on are by no means frequent, but rare occurrences that will add variety and adrenaline to my job. By the end of my F1 year I may actively look forward to them, the chance to take charge of an acute clinical situation until senior help arrives. Those situations may be where I learn some of the most valuable and valued lessons and experiences of my F1 year.

The fear which I so often referred to is completely natural and, in my opinion, healthy. It is wanting to do the best for my patients and not to let them down. In short it is to try and help people like Mr R in any way and to do my job as well as I can.

A dying lesson

Once you learn how to die, you learn how to live. (Morrie Schwartz)

It is 9 o'clock in the morning on my third day of shadowing the PRHO. The past two days have been filled with secretarial-type jobs with the odd phlebotomy and cannulation. I expected today to be no different. I was standing around the file trolley and while the PRHO was briefing me about the jobs that needed to be done today, I sneaked in a quick yawn. While the rest of the ward seemed to be bright and awake, I, having been on take the night before, felt that the most appropriate place for me right now was to be tucked up nice and warm under my duvet. We were interrupted once by the sister and another time by the PRHO's bleep going off. As she went to answer it, I arched my back in an attempt to jump-start the tired muscles. I felt strangely proud to be standing here, looking oh so important with my stethoscope around my neck, pen in hand and a million things to get done – a very important person. Over the past two days, it had been nice to have nurses mistake me for a doctor, patients thanking me for my help and strangers in the cafeteria looking at me with some form of adulation (or they appeared to be looks of adulation!). But for passing finals, I thought, 'Hey, I could do this, piece of cake!' It was in the middle of this little grandiose self-delusion that I got the true jump-start that would wake me up forever.

A nurse had appeared from one of the side rooms and she was frantically gesturing for help. I happily volunteered myself. She said that she had put out a call for the crash team and that the patient inside had had a cardiac arrest. At that moment I had the 'deer in the headlights' response – I froze. In my short time involved with the medical profession I had witnessed, in total, two cardiac arrests. I have had my intermediate life-support course as well as an advanced life-support course. However, nothing would have prepared me for today. My PRHO was nowhere to be seen, and the nurse started to point towards the crash trolley and indicated that I should bring it as quickly as possible. In the room, another nurse was removing the headboard from the bed, and I tried manoeuvring the defibrillator through the doors. No one ever told me it was that heavy! Most of everything else was hazy. The nurse started performing basic life support while I started doing chest compressions. There was a sense of urgency in everyone's expression; however, we all endeavoured to stay calm. It seemed like an eternity before the crash team arrived, and with them came expert help. The anaesthetist took charge immediately and the atmosphere became more sedate.

With my head pumped full of adrenaline, I started to look at the patient for the first time. He was 89 years old, bald and had a distended abdomen. His colour had changed from pink to blue and while I was kneeling above him, I noticed how hopeless he looked. By this time, he had been intubated and from my bird's eye view position, one of the doctors was looking for a vein, another preparing the adrenaline. A small group of spectators had formed, encompassing some of my fellow students and nurses. I was beginning to feel tired from doing chest compressions, but I felt that I had to go on. Finally, a voice behind me offered to relieve me. Beads of sweat had formed on my brow, and as I stood to one side I realised that I was breathing very heavily. After a couple of minutes, I resumed chest compressions, with a renewed strength. His chest seemed much more flaccid; it seemed that what we were doing was futile. Half an hour had passed, and the anaesthetist turned to all of us and suggested we stop. I was silent. A big part of me wanted to say that I could go on. I must go on. However, we all nodded. As I stepped off the bed, I looked at the ECG screen. He was in asystole. The clock on the wall said it was 9.43.

On the first day of the course, we had several tutorials regarding what we thought the responsibilities of a PRHO were. Several themes were identified, with the most important being patient care. To me, this concept was the most terrifying. As a rookie doctor, I expected myself to be making a number of mistakes with the hope that from each disaster comes knowledge and experience. My fear was that a second chance might just mean a second try to make the same mistake again. Superimpose that on the fragility of human life and you get insecurity, sweaty palms and added anxiety.

The issues of cardiac arrest and many other acute emergencies play in my mind consistently. As a medical student, you are shielded from the horrors of emergency medicine. It becomes more of a spectator sport; one where we can cast our eyes away when needed or bathe in its glory. The burden of disappointment, the weight of incompetence or the pressures of dealing with real-life patients and knowing that what you do may have severe consequences hardly exists for us. Reflection and self-appraisal were less important and the major preoccupations were with the multiple-choice questions and end-of-year OSCEs. The death of the 'patient in the side room' changed this for me; let me tell you how.

9 am

I was tired. Not looking forward to another ward round – more paperwork, more jobs to do. My mind was wandering. How will I cope when I have to do this for real? The notes I make are important. Listening to the patient must be the priority. How else would you know what to do next? Therefore, I should not let my mind wander. I should ask for help if needed.

9.10 am

I am the second person at the scene of a cardiac arrest. I know that as a PRHO the likelihood of me being the first person at such a scenario is fairly high. What seemed to be a slow-paced morning turned out to be a script from *ER*. This could happen at any time of the day and any time of the night, in any room, in any corridor. Will I know what to do? Five years of medical training, life-support courses and mental preparation – will I be able to apply myself? Will I be able to stay calm and focused especially when tired? After all, what I do now may alter the life of my patient. I should never be afraid to ask for help. Experienced professionals surround me.

9.15 am

Help arrives (thank goodness). Someone assumes the role of team leader. I am now part of the team, and our one goal is to help this patient to the best of our ability. I enjoyed doing chest compressions, obviously when put into context. I feel it is the vital part of the process, but yet, when deconstructed, it is the least difficult. Therefore I am not only part of the team, but am performing a vital role. However, in my haste and nervousness, am I perfusing the patient adequately without causing further damage? When I reach a more senior stage, would I be able to cannulate the patient or intubate? Could I be the team leader and would I be able to communicate my intentions well and be open to suggestions? I did get tired doing chest compressions, and in such circumstances where aid is easily available. I should recognise my limitations and ask for help. As a PRHO, a major role is that of a student and I should take advantage of different situations to acquire new clinical, communication and organisational skills because these are invaluable.

9.43 am

No cause for the cardiac arrest could be identified. With the agreement of all involved – me the medical student, the doctors, the nurses and the resuscitation team – resuscitation is discontinued. We worked as a team and therefore we should decide the outcome as a team. This, I believe, would optimise patient care and should be applied to all aspects of his/her care. However, what if I had said that we should not stop? Another three minutes, another dose of adrenaline and maybe his circulation would return. Did I partake in an effort to save a patient or was I involved in killing him? Where do we draw the line between beneficence and non-maleficence? The team leader thanks the team for their efforts and everyone, but for two nurses, leaves to continue with their busy schedules. I walk back to my trolley, still silent. I do not know whether I should talk or cry. No one else says anything. The PRHO whose care the patient was under fills in the paperwork. The nurses clean up the room, and the patient is tucked beneath his blanket as if sleeping. The door closes and life goes on.

10.15 am

The daughter and son-in-law of the deceased patient arrive. A nurse greets them and with tears in their eyes they enter the room. The PRHO follows. This would be me in less than six months. Would I be able to break the bad news? Will I be able to rely on my compassion and years of communication training to ease the pain for his relatives? If I feel the repercussions of the event, will I be able to seek help?

11 am

The room is empty. Nurses remake the bed and a new patient is soon propped up on a pillow, reading a newspaper. I look around. A phlebotomist is doing her rounds, nurses are at their station talking, I am standing with my PRHO near a bed taking a history. As we walk past the side room, my PRHO whispers softly that that was the first cardiac arrest she has witnessed as a doctor. I see her eyes well up with tears. I am relieved. It was not just me who needed to talk. I can be human.

The next step

Thinking back on my experiences during the week of PRHO shadowing, I find myself still numbed by the 'patient in the side room'. I felt that he was the culmination of all my fears and worries of working as doctor. Overall I felt that there were two major learning points. First, medicine is an unpredictable profession, simply because it deals with life. Nothing in life is guaranteed and therefore we have to do our best to be prepared. A PRHO forms part of a much larger team, and his/her involvement, regardless of how insignificant, will always have consequences. The steep learning curve, whose ultimate goal is teaching us how to be prepared, is therefore not one confined only to clinical competence, but to all elements of patient care. Second, we are all but witnesses to the cycle of life. It is the observation of oneself, regardless of the trials and tribulations, that allows us to become better active observers. Self-appraisal and the recognition of learning needs and limitations are the tools that help us to become better doctors.

As a naïve medical student, I walk around hoping that the walls of an institution will protect me forever. Learning is taught didactically; failed exams can be retaken. As I approach the next step with much excitement and nervousness, I realise that I am far from being a doctor. For it is not what is written in textbooks that counts, it is the experience – both good and bad. Right now, I just cannot wait to start experiencing.

> And let today embrace the past with remembrance
> And the future with longing. (Kahlil Gibran)

Rest in peace, Mr Fisher

I played nervously with my stethoscope as I walked in. The lights were off and the ward was filled with a cold blue light that made the almost empty room feel like a morgue. Outside a car drove past, making the windows rattle like the teeth of a shivering skeleton. A shiver ran down my spine. Only one bed in the ward was occupied (another Norwalk outbreak); a white-haired crinkle-faced man sat bathed in the bluish glow of a television, ignoring what he knew was in the bed next to him behind the curtains. He glanced up as he heard my shoes click on the tiles and looked away quickly – he knew why I was there.

Either I was early or Sarah was late. I was doing this as a favour and to prepare for next year; she hadn't wanted to do this alone and I wouldn't have wanted to either. It seemed foolish for a qualified doctor to feel anxious about being alone with a dead body, but it was almost a ritual to do this in pairs. Given the choice I wouldn't be here at all, and I was close to leaving by the time Sarah arrived with an unspoken apology in her nervous smile.

Sarah drew back the curtains and we walked inside, my stomach knotted with a quiet sense of dread. On the bed lay Clive Fisher, his eyes closed and his hands folded across his chest. I liked Clive; he he a ready smile and bright blue eyes that would light up every time he told one of his bad jokes. He was middle-aged, about 50, and his wife was sitting downstairs in reception calmly talking to nurses with red-rimmed eyes; Mr Fisher had been unofficially dead for just over an hour. A cough from Sarah told me it was time to begin, and with two gloved fingers I felt awkwardly for a pulse in his neck.

His skin was cold and his body lifeless and limp. Bending over the bed I could see his once-rosy cheeks had faded to grey. There was no steady throb of pulse and with quivering hands I filled my ears with the numb metal of my stethoscope, listening for a last impossible sign that he was still breathing. With a crack and a whisper my stethoscope burst into life and I leapt backwards in shock before I could stop myself. I knew it was only the stethoscope amplifying a brush across his skin, but for that brief moment Mr Fisher was alive and about to leap from the bed. Sarah smirked at me and began to check Mr Fisher's eyes.

With a gloved finger she drew back his eyelids, exposing two glassy eyes staring into infinity. What was he looking at, I mused absent-mindedly? Could he see through the cracked paint and grey concrete of the ceiling to heaven? Sarah took out her pen torch and shone a light into them. Could he see the light, I wondered. If he were to suddenly return to the world of the living, would he tell of travelling down a tunnel towards a blinding light? I pinched myself, and sternly told myself not to be absurd. We were here to certify the death of a patient, not to waste our time asking ourselves senseless questions. Mr Fisher is dead, and, however much I had liked him, this would solve nothing.

From outside the curtain I heard the volume of the television increase. The patient in the bed next to Mr Fisher knew he was dead; he knew what we were doing, we knew what we were doing, and it seemed that nobody wanted to acknowledge the fact. With a sigh I pushed the stethoscope back across his chest and listened intently for a heartbeat. It all seemed so unnecessary. His skin was cold, his eyes were fixed and, in short, he was dead. Who were we trying to prove it to? Sarah knew he was dead, I knew he was dead, perhaps the only person who didn't was Mr Fisher, who lay there contentedly, gazing earnestly at the cracks in the ceiling. Mr Fisher was officially dead. We had written up our notes and findings and had concluded the obvious. With a flourish Sarah signed her name on the death certificate. Underneath the line I read the legend 'May they rest in peace' and it made me think. To Sarah he may have just been another patient, but to me he was a friendly man who had been condemned to death by a weak heart. I closed my eyes for a second.

Mr Fisher; portly Mr Fisher with smiling eyes and a ready grin, rest in peace.

Glossary

A&E	Accident and emergency department, formerly known as casualty
ABC	Airway, breathing, circulation, checklist for initial assessment of a patient
ABG	Arterial blood gases
ABPI	Ankle brachial pressure index, a way of assessing disease of the blood vessels in the leg
AIDS	Acquired immune deficiency syndrome. The illness resulting from infection with the human immuno-deficiency virus
ALS	Acute life-support course
ATLS	Acute trauma life-support course
bd	Drugs given twice a day
BIPAP	Biphasic positive airways pressure, a form of ventilation, i.e. helping a patient to breath
BNF	*British National Formulary*, formulary of all drugs available
BP	Blood pressure
CCU	Coronary care unit
Cheese and onion	*Oxford Handbook of Medicine*. Beloved of medical students, similar colouring to a packet of cheese and onion crisps
COPD	Chronic obstructive pulmonary disease
CPAP	Continuous positive airways pressure, a form of ventilation, i.e. helping a patient to breath
CT	Computed tomography scan
CV	Curriculum vitae
CVP	Central venous pressure
CXR	Chest x-ray
D&V	Diarrhoea and vomiting
DNAR	Do not attempt resuscitation order
ECG	Electrocardiogram or heart tracing
EMI	Nursing home for the elderly, mentally infirm or ill
ENT	Ear, nose and throat
ERCP	Endoscopic retrograde cholangiopancreatogram, a means of imaging the liver, gall bladder and pancreas
F1	Foundation Programme doctor year 1
GCS	Glasgow Coma Scale, used to assess conscious level
GMC	General Medical Council
GP	General practitioner
Hb	Haemoglobin, level may fall in anaemia or with bleeding
HIV	Human immuno-deficiency virus
ICU or ITU	Intensive care/treatment unit
ILS	Intermediate life support course
IV	Intravenous
LFTs	Liver function tests
MAU	Medical Admissions Unit/Medical Assessment Unit
MBChB or MBBS	Bachelor of Medicine and Surgery

MDT	Multi-disciplinary team
MI	Myocardial infarction or heart attack
MRSA	Multiresistant staphylococcus aureus, a bacteria causing infection which is resistant to standard antibiotics
NG tube	Nasogastric tube
NHS	National Health Service
Obs	Observations, recording of pulse, blood pressure and temperature
od	Drugs given once daily
On call	Providing emergency cover for the wards
On take	Taking emergency admissions
OT	Occupational therapist
OSCEs	Objective structured clinical examinations
PEEP	Positive end expiratory pressure, a form of ventilation, i.e. helping a patient to breathe
Phlebotomist	Member of staff who takes blood when patients need investigations
Physio	Physiotherapist
PR	Per rectum, rectal examination
PRHO	Pre-registration house officer
'Rellies'	Shorthand for relatives
Retinopathy	Pathology of the retina often seen in people with diabetes
Sats	Saturations, indicating the level of oxygen in the blood
SAU	Surgical admissions unit
Schwann-Ganz	A special intravenous line to measure central venous pressure
SHO	Senior house officer
Sinus rhythm	Normal heart rhythm
Sphygmomanometer	Used to measure blood pressure
TTOs/TTAs	Drugs to take out or away, the drugs a patient goes home from hospital with
U&Es	Urea and electrolytes, a measure of the patient's fluid balance and kidney function
Venflons	Name of an intravenous cannula used to give intravenous fluids and drugs
VF	Ventricular fibrillation, a life-threatening abnormal heart rhythm
VT	Ventricular tachycardia, a life-threatening abnormal heart rhythm

Index